OXFORD MEDICAL PUBLICATIONS

Primary care for older people

Primary Care
for Older
People

STEVE ILIFFE AND VARI DRENNAN

Department of Primary Care and Population Sciences
Royal Free and UCL Medical School

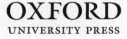
OXFORD
UNIVERSITY PRESS

B S

OXFORD
UNIVERSITY PRESS

Great Clarendon Street, Oxford OX2 6DP

Oxford University Press is a department of the University of Oxford.
It furthers the University's objective of excellence in research, scholarship,
and education by publishing worldwide in

Oxford New York

Athens Auckland Bangkok Bogota Bombay Buenos Aires Calcutta
Cape Town Dar es Salaam Delhi Florence Hong Kong Istanbul
Karachi Kuala Lumpur Madrid Melbourne Mexico City Mumbai
Nairobi Paris San Paulo Singapore Taipei Tokyo Toronto Warsaw

and associated companies in
Berlin Ibadan

Oxford is a registered trade mark of Oxford University Press
in the UK and in certain other countries

Published in the United States
by Oxford University Press Inc., New York

© S. Iliffe and V. Drennan, 2000

A catalogue record for this book is available from the British Library

Data available

Library of Congress Cataloging in Publication Data

Iliffe, Steve.
Primary care for older people / Steve Iliffe and Vari Drennan.
p. cm. — (Oxford general practice series ; no. 44)
Includes bibliographical references and index.
1. Aged—Medical care. 2. Primary care (Medicine)
I. Drennan, Vari II. Title. III. Series.
RC952 .I43 2000   618.97—dc21   00-038592
ISBN 019 262951 4

Typeset by
J&L Composition Ltd, Filey, North Yorkshire
Printed in Great Britain
on acid-free paper by
Biddles Ltd, Guildford & King's Lynn

CONTENTS

Coming into Eighty

Coming into eighty
I slow my ship down
For safe landing.
It has been battered,
One sail torn, the rudder
Sometimes wobbly.
We are hardly a glorious sight.
It has been a long voyage
Through time, travail and triumph,
Eighty years
Of learning what to be
And how to become it.

One day the ship will decompose
And then what will become of me?
Only a breath
Gone into nothingness
Alone
Or a spirit of air and fire
Set free?
Who knows?

Greet us at landfall
The old ship and me,
But we can't stay anchored.
Soon we must set sail
On the last mysterious voyage
Everybody takes
Toward death.
Without my ship here,
Wish me well.

May Sarton
Coming into Eighty and Earlier Poems
The Women's Press Ltd, London 1995

INTRODUCTION

The population is ageing, but so is the health service. This book is intended to rejuvenate primary care, so that it can cope with the demands of a growing cohort of older people. We have written it at a time when the structure of the National Health Service is changing yet again, threatening practitioners with more wearisome jargon and regulations, but also offering us enormous opportunities to improve our knowledge and our work. The flirtation with market mechanisms in the NHS is ending, and the processes of clinical governance is drawing general practice, community nursing, and social care closer together than they have ever been before. This is the opportunity of a professional lifetime to turn the rhetoric of 'seamless care' into the reality of primary care that is holistic, systematic, and evidence-based.

The first beneficiaries of this should be older people because the ageing population carries the burden of illness and disability, poses the most complex diagnostic and therapeutic problems, and reaps the most benefit from medical and nursing care. When we listen to our older patients, and react to their problems, we have to understand the past and present psychology and sociology of our time, as well as the intricacies of ageing physiology and anatomy. That is why we make no apologies for our bias towards understanding the past, in the hopes of not repeating its errors. Similarly we do not avoid the details of diseases and disabilities because those who cannot grasp why older people may fall, or become depressed, or respond so well to ACE inhibitors, will not cope successfully with the demographic shift of the early 21st century.

Since people in old age represent all the diversity of the rest of the adult population, their expectations and use of primary health care services are equally diverse. As with the rest of the population, the influences on health and well-being are multifactorial and the provision of treatment, cure and care in illness, disability, and dying are not the sole province of one agency or grouping. This book reflects this multiplicity of perspectives on the range of situations in which primary health care participates – a continuum from anticipatory care, health promotion, through to acute care, rehabilitation, continuing care, and care of people who are dying.

In rereading the literature for this book we received a strong impression of parallel professional and system universes – a feeling that can be replicated for older people with more complex health and social problems in dealing with the services. The book is structured in such a way to encircle the clinical information within information on the infrastructures necessary for quality in health care of older people. It also places clinical information firmly within the health and social care systems, indicating the relevant social policy. The national critiques of health and social care services for older people have pointed repeatedly for the need for 'whole system' approaches. We have tried to reflect this in the structure and content of this book. If sometimes we seem critical of community nurses and general practitioners it is not because we view them from some lofty specialist perch, but because primary care practitioners have been left unaided to struggle with immensely difficult problems and not surprisingly have often failed. It is time to put that right, and we hope that through our discussion of agendas for primary care groups and primary care research networks, this book will contribute to doing so.

We provide a pathway through the book – from the individual to the collective, from the historical to the future. We focus first on evidence and information related to the care of the individual, then move to approaches in the provision of care at a team and PCG level. We specifically draw on a historical perspective at the beginning of the book and end with planning for the future and an agenda for PCGs. Core principles that run throughout the book are the need for systematic processes in determining priorities, provision of service, and then review. We repeat these principles in the care of the individual – through advocacy of proactive case management – and in the care of the population – through advocacy of health needs assessment processes such as community-orientated primary care .

This is not a textbook of geriatric medicine and nursing – we only refer to leg ulcers to demonstrate how easily evidence-based practice can become narrow and unhelpful, and screening for prostate cancer is not mentioned at all. There are plenty of sources of technical knowledge that are better and timelier than anything we could produce, but there are few that try to give the whole picture and show how ideas fit together and help practice to change. We have chosen clinical conditions because they are so complex and baffling to practitioners – such as falls, or dementia – or neglected despite being to some extent amenable to medical intervention, such as heart disease, depression or chronic obstructive airways disease.

Nor is it our intention to provide glib, easy answers. The reality is that they do not exist, but there are many strategies which could significantly improve the nature and level of care provided for older people in primary care. Primary health care for older people in the 21st century has all the lessons of the 20th to learn from, the new technologies to address old problems, and the potential for truly creative change.

Steve Iliffe and Vari Drennan
Department of Primary Care and Population Sciences
Royal Free and UCL Medical School, London

CHAPTER ONE

Innovation in primary care for older people – what went wrong?

In 1948 the National Health Service (NHS) inherited a massive amount of unmet medical need, especially amongst the older generation that had not been the focus for pre-war efforts to improve child and maternal health, or to eradicate infectious disease.[1,2] This included a backlog of endlessly-postponed gynaecological surgery, and a cohort of old men sitting at home with catheterized bladders for want of prostate operations. The NHS made dentures for edentulous pensioners previously denied access to dental care through lack of money and a shortage of dentists, and corrected short-sightedness and cataract in the three-quarters of the population who had never had access to free ophthalmic services. It is no surprise that the first recipient generation described their NHS as 'the envy of the world', for it rewarded them for their efforts, suffering and sacrifice in wars and economic depression.

This backlog of unmet need was dealt with effectively by the NHS,[3] the principal driving force being the emergence of geriatric medicine as a speciality that could bring acute medical care and rehabilitation to a population of older people previously denied it.[4] In 1948 there were no more than half a dozen hospital physicians in Britain who had a special interest in the care of older patients, but by 1983 there were more than 500 working with multidisciplinary teams to provide acute medical care, rehabilitation, and long-term care for older people. The impact of this speciality was such that by the early seventies the predominant problem amongst older people in the community was seen to be functional loss, not undiagnosed medical problems.[5] The majority of medical problems identified by screening of older populations were either already known to the general practitioner or were not considered of major importance by the individuals concerned.[6,7] Consultation habits appeared to have changed after the establishment of a free health service, with less evidence of under-consultation by older patients,[8] and some signs that those who did not seek medical care were relatively well.[9] The impact of this change cannot be underestimated. Extensive growth of services that repaired pathologies was not a solution to problems that were as much social and psychological as organic. Heart valves damaged by rheumatic fever, vaginal

1

prolapses and cataracts were easier to put right than combinations of osteoarthritis, obesity and depressed mood, and similar complex combinations of illness and disability. General practice had a perspective on the organic, psychological and social dimensions of ill health in the last quarter of the 20th century, but for reasons that we will visit in this chapter, and review in later ones, it was not able to apply this perspective effectively.

The development of an interest in primary care for older people was less significant, and much less rapid, than the growth of geriatric medicine, but it began in the 1950s and gathered some momentum in the heyday of general practice, in the seventies and early eighties. It hinged on finding a role for primary care staff – general practitioners (GPs) and health visitors in particular – to complement that of specialist geriatric medicine. Were general practitioners simply to direct their older patients towards geriatricians, or was there some other task to perform, like preventing them from needing specialist care at all? Were health visitors to concentrate on the health of infants and preschool children, or did they have a broader remit for health promotion across all age groups?

The issue was not just how to respond to individual older patients, but how to have an impact on the whole of an ageing population. If checking every adult's blood pressure was a way to find people with hypertension, and testing all toddlers' vision and hearing a way to detect potentially remediable sensory impairment, why not apply the same principles to older age groups? Screening of whole populations, and assessment of individuals using standardized measures, were ideas that appealed to the first generation of primary care gerontologists. As we shall show, the ideas became confused in the early 1990s, and are only now becoming untangled.

Experimentation with population screening and assessment by different methods such as postal questionnaires, specialist nurses, case-finding computer software and dedicated clinics, and the search for 'at risk' groups were reflected in the debates that occurred both in the Royal College of General Practice[5] and in the Health Visitors Association [5]. Although the reporting of the approaches to primary care for older people was dominated by general practitioners, much of the actual work on the ground was pioneered by health visitors, and the underlying ideas came as much from community nursing as from medicine.[11,12]

We are not going to repeat the debates here, although they are fascinating because they were so wide-ranging and their conclusions were realistic but cautious. The lack of evidence for the effectiveness of geriatric screening should not be allowed to undermine enthusiasm for studying the best ways to provide anticipatory care for older people, but the iatrogenic risks of treating unimportant abnormalities, and of medicalizing old age, were acknowledged.[13] Brief, non-intrusive strategies for predicting functional problems during routine consultations were needed, which should be tested in randomized controlled trials, despite the methodological problems of standardizing data collection and inadequate outcome measures.[14] The preoccupation of doctors with disease to the detriment of its social consequences, the failure to take into account the adaptive powers of older people, and the tendency to underestimate the burden borne by carers were all identified as major obstacles to progress in developing more effective primary care for older people. Medical and social problems overlapped in ways that were often puzzling to clinicians, screening led to an increase in referrals to other agencies but without clear evidence of benefit in many instances, and with variations in referral rates determined as much by the referrer as by the patient's problems.[15] Finally, at risk groups proved harder to identify than anticipated, for more pathological events occurred outside the expected at risk groups than in them. At the same time health visitors were experimenting with different ways of undertaking health-promoting work with this age group, using as their inspiration models of community development and community networking. [16, 17] These approaches looked promising, precisely because they began from a social understanding of the impact of disease, and the recognition that disability is the gap between individual capability and environmental demand.

The generation of GPs and nurses who did this work introduced important ideas about how ageing in its organic, social, and psychological dimensions affected people's health, how essential multidisciplinary teamwork was to providing appropriate care for ill older people,[18] and ultimately how networking with community-based agencies was a more useful model than referral to specialist care.[19] This framework of thinking arose from the intellectual strengths of their disciplines, which synthesized knowledge from different domains in different ways to describe, and change, the complex environment of life in an advanced industrial society at the end of the 20th century. However, at a time when medical science was focusing with increasing intensity on experimental methods of testing new ideas, it also became a weakness.

There was no shortage of enthusiasm and hope for development. The programme of the British Geriatric Society and the Health Visitors Association (paraphrased and slightly shortened, Box 1.1) was set out in a positive manifesto for a new primary care geriatric assessment service. No one working in primary care now is likely to recognize much of it in existence in their locality, although many might welcome its appearance.

Science as experiments

Generalist approaches based on biopsychosocial models might make sense to practitioners in the community, but they could only be tested using experimental methods when broken down into their components. The problems of confusing clinical epidemiology and general practice were clear to those involved in innovation and service development.[13] Although it was obvious that an 84-year-old, housebound widow should get closer attention than a married and mobile 71-year-old, hidden problems in people of apparently low risk occurred often enough to warrant consideration, whilst those with greatest need may neither have requested nor used help that was offered. The perception that the older patient lived within a system of relationships

Box 1.1 *Health visiting for the health of the aged – a joint policy state-ment from the British Geriatric Society and the Health Visitors Association, 1986*

- Health visitors should provide health promotion and prevention for all older people.
- Health visitors should undertake assessment of health status, plan actions to satisfy unmet needs, and liase with hospitals.
- Health visitors should develop expertise at group level, with at least one in each group specializing in working with elderly people.
- Liaison posts should be filled only by qualified community nurses.
- Liaison health visitors or nurses should have appropriate logistic support.
- Health visitors for the elderly should work to protocols for planning respite care.
- A cooperation card should be the record used by all, including informal carers.
- Every referral or admission should trigger a review of medication.
- Health visitors should be aware of the ways in which older people could be assisted with correct medication use.
- Health visitors should have access to the information they need to audit work, and should profile their neighbourhood's older population and develop agreed objectives of care.
- Each health authority should formulate a detailed policy for the health visitors working with older people.
- One health visitor should be in post for every 2000 people.
- Where health visitors work in primary care teams, the team should be involved in formulation policy.
- All health visitors should receive at least five-yearly refreshment of their knowledge and skills in relation to the care of older people.

conditioned by history had to accommodate itself to the dominant paradigm of medical science shaped by surgeons and drug therapies. The symbol of technical medicine became the randomized controlled trial (RCT), the ultimate test of effectiveness of new medicines and surgical procedures. For reasons that we must leave to the historians of medicine to explore, the RCT became the preferred technique for measuring the value of any intervention anywhere, including complex interventions in the body politic.

Almost inevitably, testing the components of screening programmes for older people through randomized trials appeared to be the logical next step for geriatricians and gerontologists. Several such trials took place in the 1980s in the UK, Denmark, and the USA. Different trials used very different interventions and outcome measures, but there are some common features:[20]

- a rise in morale amongst elderly people involved in screening programmes
- referrals to all agencies tended to increase, including to specialist medical care in some studies

- the duration of in-patient stay fell in some studies, possibly through early intervention in disease processes
- in-patient rates could increase through a greater use of respite care
- reduction in mortality did occur in some trials, perhaps for the same reason that in-patient stays declined, but not in all
- no trial up to 1990 demonstrated an improvement in older people's functional ability, and general practitioner workload only decreased in situations where alternative services were organized to bypass existing primary care services.

Testing whole models of care in systemic ways that did not rely on the experimental methods of the RCT was attempted, but produced less satisfying results that did not fit into the paradigm of experimental science (and therefore did not get published in opinion-leading scientific journals). For example, linkworker approaches that used generic workers as troubleshooters for older people, and liaison workers between agencies, revealed both the complexities of actual services and the difficulties in making them work jointly.[21] Problems whose solutions still elude us were explored a decade or two ago in small-scale, mostly descriptive studies that identified the importance of older people's information needs,[22] common record systems across disciplines,[23] autonomy and independence,[24] and liaison between primary care professionals and with hospitals.[25] Community-orientated developments in health visitor services for older people were numerous,[26] occurring in inner-city areas as well as in the leafy shires,[27] and were in places subject to rigorous study.[28] This did not guarantee their survival and progress any more than it did for innovation in general practice.

Complex interventions in heterogeneous populations are difficult, perhaps impossible, to test in randomized controlled trials, but for a time such trials were the only form of testing that was accepted within scientific medicine as being a reliable pointer for service development. Whatever the merits of the randomized trial as an experimental technique, medical science must be limited in its comprehension of complex situations if it has no other methods available to it that allow practitioners to decide on what they should do, with real patients, in real life. We are now at the end of a phase of scientific thinking dominated by an intellectual monoculture, and a variety of alternative ways of thinking and studying change are emerging that may allow a second generation of primary care gerontologists to have an impact on the health of older people.

This is the dilemma that the early practitioners of primary care for older people had to face in the seventies and eighties. Their disciplines did not have any methods of evaluating the impact of their work that matched the experimental design in ways that would satisfy managers and payers who were increasingly interested in the certainties of a clear, unambiguous result. Such methods do exist, and we will discuss them in more detail in Chapter 11 when considering commissioning services for older populations, but they were not contenders in medicine in the eighties. Neither general practice nor nursing had an intellectual background and the kind of academic critical mass that could go beyond conceptualizing reality in psychosociobiological terms to evaluating psychosociobiological interventions, perhaps because both had grown out of hospital disciplines, were relative newcomers to science in any form, and had weak links with those disciplines which might have helped – psychology and sociology. Without translating their complex conceptual framework into concrete training programmes, innovative GPs and community nurses could only remain marginal to the process of primary care development. This proved particularly damaging for community nursing, especially for health visitors, whose *actual* involvement with the older population declined almost as fast as innovation grew.[29]

What might have happened had general practice and community nursing had a stronger academic basis for their work? We can only speculate with all the advantages of hindsight, but learning some lessons from this might also help us plan ahead for the next wave of innovation in care for older people that primary care commissioning could promote. Where better to start a speculative history of primary care as a social science than with the lessons to be learned from older people themselves?

Ageing, health, and illness

When do people become old? In one American study 80% of those aged 60–69 rejected the terms 'old' or 'elderly' for themselves, and even a third of those aged 80 or older thought that 'middle-aged' was a correct description of their status.[30] The experience of ageing is tightly bound to physical and social functioning. Six factors determine the transition to old age:

(1) physical health problems
(2) changes in social role
(3) retirement
(4) chronological age
(5) restrictions in physical activity
(6) the illness or death of a spouse.

The first two factors appear to carry most weight for most of us. Those with perceived good health, or with high activity levels, continue to view themselves as middle-aged. Sudden changes in health, like a stroke or a myocardial infarction, may be the transition to old age, especially if their consequences alter social relationships and activities, whilst slower changes, like reduced exercise tolerance, may indicate a process of ageing rather than a transition.

Mr A. had a stroke affecting the left side of his body not long after his 74th birthday, and within a few weeks of moving from a seaside town to a new flat in the city which he had left 30 years before. The woman with whom he had lived for 10 years left him the next day, saying that she could not care for him. After a brief hospital admission where rehabilitation was started he made a good functional recovery, aided by visits from the community physiotherapist, modification to his (ground-floor) flat by the occupational therapist from social services, and home-help support from social services.

He remained distraught at the loss of the woman he still loved, and frustrated by his inability to do all the things he needed and wanted to do around the flat and in his tiny garden. During visits to his GP he would sometimes weep copiously, but he always refused any medication for his depressed mood, sleeplessness, and lack of energy. Although he often said that he saw no point in going on, he slowly became more socially active, finally joining a senior citizens' exercise class at the local gym and a luncheon club where he got 'good food and some company'. He said 'they are all old fogeys, but so am I now'.

Changes in social activity and status are potent indicators of the transition for some. The generation of women who were never formally employed outside the home, except perhaps during wartime, may attach no meaning to 'retirement', but if their husbands survived the events of mid-century their own retirement from paid work was their exit from the world of financial independence to that of dependency. For older women the death of their spouse in old age, or the arrival of grandchildren, might be markers of transition.[31]

Mrs B. worked very hard for over 30 years in a famous department store, commuting to work on a scooter in all weathers, but had looked forward to retirement because of her passion for a famous singer. She not only went to every concert he gave, even if it meant travelling abroad, but ran an international fan club. On top of this she managed a large house with several rooms which she let to lodgers, and looked after her husband, a disabled war veteran some 10 years her senior. Retirement did not produce the pleasure she had expected because she developed diabetes and asthma soon after ceasing work and her husband had the first of three heart attacks, the last of which was fatal. Left alone in her early seventies she wondered whether she was fit enough to ride her scooter and go to concerts anymore at the age of 73, although she had had no doubt about this when she was 72 and her husband was still alive.

The ideas about health and illness held by the generations now entering their seventies or eighties do not always match contemporary attitudes, particularly those that are the conventional wisdom of health and social care professionals. Explanations of health and illness used by any individual may also change as time passes and circumstances alter. Those who have a chronic disease or long-standing disability are less likely to define health as the absence of illness than their healthier peers. Instead they may define health (and their own healthiness) pragmatically as the ability to do things, or to maintain relationships (particularly to help others), or the experience of well-being and contentedness.[32] There appears to be a menu of eight important explanatory models from which older people can choose to create a personal 'guide to action':[33]

(1) the body as a machine – doctors understand the body in this way, and if things go wrong with it, modern medicine can do something about the fault

7

(2) the body under siege – external events, pressures, and threats challenge the body continuously, and heredity may undermine it too, but there is no moral blame attached to illnesses that these factors induce

(3) the health promotion model – good health is a matter of maintaining a healthy lifestyle

(4) inequality of access – ill health is related to limited access to resources and advantages, for which others are to blame

(5) The cultural critique – the unequal distribution of power and knowledge is more important than the unequal distribution of resources

(6) God's will – health is the gift of the good and a reward for good living, whilst ill health is a sign of, or punishment, for moral lapses

(7) willpower matters – mind can overcome matter, and bodies are self-healing

(8) robust individualism – the individual must choose, and live with the consequences of their choices.

Everyone working with the present older generation has encountered all of these perceptions influencing the ways in which patients accept or reject diagnoses or treatments, respond to symptoms or ignore them, and adopt or avoid different ways of behaving with a view to altering their state of health. What may surprise professionals who see later life as being a phase of life with no future, when all that can be achieved has been, is the apparent increase in health-promoting activities engaged in after the age of 60, by both men and women.[32] Figure 1.1 shows the percentage of older people from different age groups who describe themselves as being engaged in health-promoting activities (particularly walking, gardening, and attention to a healthy diet).[34]

The implications for professionals working with older populations are clear. Health promotion initiatives of certain kinds – especially around physical activity and food – may be well received by, and effective for, individuals who have strong beliefs in the appropriateness of exercise and healthy eating, whilst those initiatives that are perceived as faddish rather than commonsense will be rejected by critical thinkers who are both experienced and scathing in their judgements.

Whilst conventional wisdom describes the current cohort of older people as relatively undemanding, uncritical, and uncomplaining, the reality is less benign. For example, the report of the contradictory and heterogeneous but fiercely held views elicited in recent interviews with working-class pensioners on a single housing estate in the North East makes sobering reading for primary care professionals.[35] Their views of health and health care included the following ideas:

- 'greedy doctors at the top'
- the government is not responsible
- the 'undeserving poor' will not change their lifestyles
- poverty and unemployment cause ill health, and responsibility for these things lies with the powers that be
- medicine affiliates with powerful interests – for example, individualizing

Figure 1.1 *Types of activities engaged in by older people.*[34]

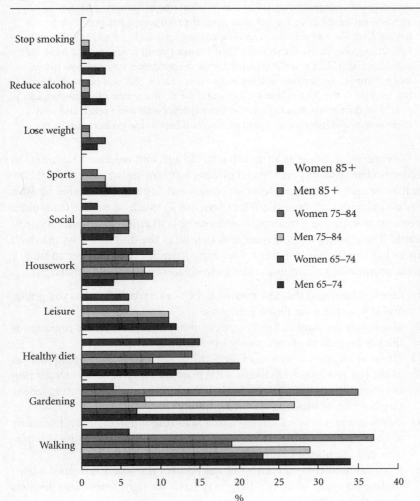

health care obscures inequalities in health
- expert knowledge can be challenged from the basis of experience
- alternative medicine is useful (if you can afford it)
- medical practitioners purposefully disempower patients by claiming expertise over the body
- age barriers to health care are unacceptable
- doctors should not exploit gender inequalities to maintain power and control
- technical rationality that is concerned with measurable outcomes but not with absolute values is wrong.

Mrs C. was very deaf, and despite wearing apparently well-tuned hearing aids, shouted very loudly. Consultations with her were slow and often punctuated by exchanges of written messages. She was 91 when one of her sons – himself in his sixties – brought her to see her new general practitioner, her previous doctor having died. She had varicose eczema, spreading up both legs from ankle to mid-calf. 'It's terribly itchy', she shouted, 'and I cannot stand it any more. I must see a skin specialist.' Her new GP explained what the condition was, and how to control it. 'You get thrown on the scrap heap when you are old,' was her reply, looking intently at the doctor, 'but I won't stand for it. You're not a fundholder, are you?' Her doctor was able to deny the latter charge, with some relief, and after a three-way negotiation she accepted some emollients to use on her skin.

We experience illness as a transition to old age, and redefine healthiness to accommodate disability or chronic disease, but how do we deal with disease itself as we age? If older people are so committed to being and staying healthy, why do primary care professionals experience so much resistance from older people to investigation, treatments and attempts to ameliorate disability or ill health? The answers to these questions may lie in the different ways in which illness has significance for those who experience it. There appear to be five broad assumptions about how older individuals can cope with illness:[36]

(1) illness is managed through normal living – everyday life keeps you going, and if you stop your illness gets worse
(2) illness as a constant struggle – determination not to become impaired is the key ingredient of this coping mechanism
(3) illness as an alternative way of life – this is not a common coping mechanism, but it allows individuals with poor mobility or vision to develop new behaviours that circumvent their disabilities, such as adopting sedentary hobbies or listening to 'talking books'
(4) illness as a loss to be endured – individuals respond to their limitations by abandoning previous activities and interests, stoically and without bitterness and resentment, but with resignation
(5) illness as a relief from effort – illness releases the individual from a continuing struggle, although they may have strongly ambivalent feelings about this escape.

These assumptions can be combined into complex motives for action or inaction in the face of illness and disability. The first and second assumptions can be combined to make ill health a test of achievement, or even an occupation in which the individual struggles with or against illness but is always preoccupied with it. The first and fourth assumptions combine to make illness a destroyer, or less threateningly a place of exile that still challenges the self. Assumptions four and five fit together to produce disengagement, and bring us back to the belief that in our later life we are living on borrowed time. Disengagement, first from social and family responsibilities and work, then from personal and home care tasks, and finally from life itself, is a course which many follow and as a model of ageing it has had a powerful impact on practice, stressing the importance of psychological adjustment. It is not an accurate description of the ways in which the majority of the older population lives and dies, although it may correspond to the experience that professionals in primary and social care have of those older people who are to a lesser or greater extent dependent upon them.

It is worth considering here another theory on disengagement to inform professional practice. Social policy has provided a significant force in creating the conditions for disengagement and what has been described as 'structured dependency'. [37] The structural forces of government legislation on retirement age, state pensions levels, and married women sharing the husband's pension impact significantly on the income levels of older people. Disengagement can be construed as a consequence of low income rather than individual psychology. In this analysis, professional practice needs to consider the impact of low incomes on older people, and the potential changes in social situation, well-being, and health that might follow from an increase in income.

Just as the explanatory model of health can be changed as the individual's situation changes, so too can the coping mechanisms for illness. For the practitioner, the implication is one of understanding individual psychology in sufficient detail to be able to place each patient within a spectrum of beliefs and attitudes, so that work can be attempted with some expectation of success.

Aged 91, Mrs D. lives alone in a third-floor, one-bedroom flat in a small, relatively modern block of flats. Widowed for 20 years, she has a daughter (in her sixties) who lives 35 miles away, and one or two local friends whom she sees regularly each week. A neighbour helps her with shopping, and brings her to the practice from time to time. Travelling is a real struggle for her.

She is partially sighted (because of macular degeneration), and is just able to see the outlines of people and things, but no detail. She cannot watch television or read, but enjoys listening to the radio and talking books, even though she is moderately deaf. She had a myocardial infarction seven years ago, and has had cardiac failure since, causing progressively worsening exertional breathlessness and swelling of the ankles and calves.

One particularly wet day in November she requests a house call from her doctor, who goes anticipating further deterioration in her condition. 'I'm remarkably well,' she says, 'but I wanted a flu jab – I hope you've brought one. And can I have one of those new ones against pneumonia.' She takes the opportunity of the visit to ask for her GP's support in pressing for more home care from social services because of her worsening vision and declining ability to prepare food and drink. She disarms her GP's irritation at being called out for something that he felt could be dealt with differently by demonstrating a sensor that she has bought to fit over the rim of a mug to signal when it is full enough, which her doctor has never seen before.

Pessimism about the value of work with older people is widespread in both primary and social care,[38] translating into self-imposed limitations in effort, inaction and a lack of creativity in responding to problems.[39] It could also be argued that this has influenced service developments and priorities. The rhetoric of the profession of health visiting in working with people from 'the cradle to the grave' was never a reality. During this period, even though some areas developed 'geriatric visitors' (see p.4), the contact levels with people aged over 65 decreased. The failure of health visitors to develop a role with older people in the community reflected their individual pessimism about old age and the lack of a reference framework in which to construct their encounters. It partly explains their widespread absence from anticipatory care of older people,[40] outside the experimental and innovative projects described earlier in this chapter. Likewise, district nursing never responded to the exhortations of increased involvement in health promotion and anticipatory care with older people.[41] However, the expansion or reorientation of a health visiting or district nursing service also depended on the decision-making at a district or area level – either of these meant investing financially in older people rather than children or other services and therefore reflected institutional ageism as well as individual pessimism.

There appears to be a tendency for younger professionals to both overestimate their awareness of the needs of older people and their theoretical knowledge of biological, social, and psychological changes associated with later life, and to fill gaps in knowledge either with the predominantly negative stereotypes of old age current in society, or with extrapolations from their own priorities, concerns, and experiences.[42] Attempts to remedy this in social work have developed around the 'confronting ageing approach' and 'ageism awareness training', both group-work approaches that have yet to reach medicine and community nursing.

Confronting ageing requires groups to work through knowledge about real older people with whom group members have contact, as well as anticipating their own old age and exploring issues of communication, power, and collusion.[43] Ageism awareness training encourages group participants to divest themselves of contemporary adult perspectives on age by first reconsidering their own childhood before answering questions about later life:[44]

- What do you like about older people?
- What have you liked about an old person whom you know?
- What can't you stand about old people?
- What is your greatest fear about growing old (or older) or being old?
- How should life be for you, when you are old?
- What would you say to your older future self from where you stand now?
- If there were no stereotypes of old age, if you were confident and without fear, how would your relationships with older people change?

Answers to these questions then allow the group and individuals to consider how their working practices and personal relationships could be changed. Some of these changes may depend on acquiring an understanding of how important a sense of coherence is for ill or disabled people, who exist on a spectrum of health and ill health, not in one of two distinct states. (The spectrum explains why it is so hard to identify an at risk group amongst older people upon which attention can be focused.) This coherence consists of comprehensibility, meaningfulness, and manageability.[45] Comprehensibility means that each person can make sense of their situation, and requires the professional to understand the range of explanatory models available to their older patients. Meaningfulness is the emotional equivalent of comprehensibility, whilst manageability refers to the patient's ability to deal with evolving situations of illness and disability within their given resources.

The continuing evolution of training to enhance consultation skills is one of the great strengths of general practice, and inclusion of a theoretical framework based on sense of coherence and relevant to work with older patients is perfectly possible. But what about the issue of resources to match the varying needs and requirements of an ageing population? 'It's not what you've got, it's the way that you use it' may be true at times, but the material circumstances of the older generations make a huge impact on the health of older individuals, and on their families' economies. These are outside the scope of traditional medicine, even in general practice, and lie with social service departments, benefits agencies, voluntary organizations, and the efforts of individual citizens. In Chapter 2 we will comment on differences between Britain and our north European neighbours in approaches to supporting families and older people, but here we will use examples from social care in the 1970s and 1980s to shed light on the missed opportunities for anticipatory primary care for older people.

Social and health care – boundaries and territory

The development of social care for older people in the community paralleled that of geriatric medicine in hospitals, with extension of services across the whole country and the emergence of specialist expertise. Although the relationship between social circumstances – housing, income, support – and health in later life was well known to clinicians and social service workers alike, close working relationships between disciplines ostensibly concerned with the same group of people in need have always been problematic. As geriatric medicine in hospitals burgeoned, it became obvious to clinicians that discharging older patients to survive on low incomes in poor-quality accommodation was futile, yet living in relative poverty in undermaintained homes with limited amenities was a common experience for older age groups[31].

The first attempt to overcome the fragmentation of care (and address concerns about rising expenditure) was the 1974 reorganization of the NHS.[46] Before 1974 the health service had three components – the hospitals, local authority health services (including district nurses, health visitors, home helps, and ambulance services all organized in the Medical Officers of Health division), and the independently contracted services of general practice, dentists, opticians, and pharmacists. One of the backdrops for this reorganization, and that of the local authorities in the same period, was the embryonic policy agenda of increased levels of care in the community rather than large institutional settings. The 1974 reorganization of the NHS took community nursing away from local government and merged it with the hospital system, whilst social services were placed firmly under the control of local government.

After 1974, geriatric medicine in hospitals, and community nursing organized from hospitals, both developed working relationships with local government social services, but they were never able to merge into unified multidisciplinary teams. Two policy options that might have allowed this – for the hospital service to absorb local government's personal social services, or to be absorbed by local government to create integrated services – were never on the political agenda for the NHS, which tended to favour pragmatic 'second best' approaches[3] that emphasized joint working between autonomous structures. Joint working was not always easy, but social services did expand to provide rehabilitation and support for older people in the community on a scale that was significant, if never on the scale of other welfare states (see Chapter 2). Personal social services for community-dwelling older people were widespread enough to provide some comfort in later life for many frail individuals, and were sensitive enough to an individual citizen's needs to allow for, and respond to, the quality of relationships between family members in providing services. Davies' analysis of the factors determining use of social services home care by older people revealed that the presence or absence of confiding relationships, and the declared motivation of the principal carer, were as significant as the level of disability, the presence of incontinence or confusion, or measurable functional loss.[47] Social care became a kind of state-provided consumer good for older people in need, even if it was never available as a citizen's right and was not intended as a substitute for institutional care. All this began to change in the eighties, as we shall show in Chapter 2.

What was true for community nursing about joint working with social care did not necessarily apply to general practice. Relationships between general practice and social services were particularly difficult, partly because of the different working cultures of the two disciplines.[48] Nevertheless, joint working began to have some impact and relationships began to improve in the seventies, with attachment of social workers to practices being the dominant model up until the mid-1980s. However, there is some evidence that such attachments worked against needs of older people because practice-attached social workers became involved in the demand-led culture of general practice and received referrals of a younger, more psychologically troubled patient group.[49] This phase of joint working came to an end in the late eighties because of financial problems in local government, and attached social workers were withdrawn from general practice, only to be reintroduced on a limited scale after the implementation in 1993 of the Community Care Act. More recently, a new Secretary of State for Health has called for the 'tearing down of the Berlin Wall' between health and social care, without specifying how this can be done and what the subsequent professional topography might look like.

Table 1.1 is derived from descriptions of pre-Community Care Act generic social worker attachment schemes and attempts to compare them with 'normal care.'[48] It is an amalgamation of several different studies. Nearly half of all patients referred to practice-based social workers were young and for two-thirds of them their primary problem was psychological. This pattern did not reflect the types of patients GPs would normally refer to a social services

Table 1.1 *Social worker attachments in general practices compared with standard services*

Client type	GP referrals to social services departments (%)	GP referrals to practice-based social worker (%)	All referrals to social services department(%)
Age < 45	less than 30	47	39
Age > 65	76	30	37
Per cent female	67	70	58
Owner/occupier	55	19	21
Council housing	31	42	27
Private rented	21	37	32
Practical problem	83	32	61
Psychological problem	17	66	22

department, 76% of whom were over 65 and over 80% of whom had primarily a practical problem. Neither did it reflect the overall referral pattern to social services from any source, where again most people referred or referring themselves had primarily a practical problem.

Table 1.1 suggests that the types of cases referred to attached social workers were notcomparable with those usually referred from other channels, and it seems that attached social workers may have been filling a counselling role within the practices. While this was important for the practices, it was costly for social services, reduced the social work role with older people, and may have contributed to the decision to withdraw social workers from practices in the 1980s. It also underlines the perceived role of social care as reactive rather than proactive, solving problems rather than preventing them.

While social workers will almost certainly have some knowledge of how GPs work based on their own experience as patients, the reverse is unlikely to be true. General practitioners are largely ignorant of social workers' working practices and training requirements. For example, in 1986 only 20% of GPs working in training practices in Norfolk thought social workers needed any form of higher education and only 25% thought their work usefully involved their clients' emotional or relationship problems.[50] Morris,[51] a GP in Devon, noticed during negotiations with the local social services department that there was even a language barrier; to him, an urgent referral meant something that needed immediate attention, whereas to the social services team it meant something that needed attention within two days.

This difference in the time-frame of working is one of several cultural differences that are summarized in Table 1.2.[52] While many of the differences are less marked now than they were 15 years ago, one finding in particular seems

Table 1.2 *Cultural differences in the working practices of general practitioners and social workers*

General practitioner	Social worker
Older	Younger
More often male	More often female
Leads team – as patient's advocate should not relinquish control, leads to demands for services for patient rather than requests for assessment	Team member – taught to work in egalitarian way with other agencies, certainly not to see GP in leadership role
Faster time-frame of working	Slower time-frame of working
Well respected, old profession	Less well respected, newer profession
Medical model – focuses only on individual to explain and solve problems	Social model – sees source of problem in the enviroment and orientates intervention beyond the individual

to help explain some of the still-current difficulties: action versus holding orientation. Medical training focuses on swift decision-making to enable competent handling of emergency situations. Social workers are taught that better decisions are made if a situation is contained until the perceptions and feelings of all concerned are clarified

The cultural differences in working practices may help to explain why the social services–primary care interface has traditionally been so problematic. However, different cultural values are not the only barrier. Poor communications help to maintain the lack of understanding between the professions of each other's role and working practices. In some instances this is made worse by the blurred boundary between health and social care. The consequent inability to claim exclusive knowledge and ownership of activities between social workers, district nurses, health visitors, community psychiatric nurses, and occupational therapists leads to tensions and disputes.

Mrs E., a 77-year-old widow, annoyed her neighbours by banging on the shared wall between their terraced homes, and by denouncing them fiercely in strong and racist language from her back garden and her front doorstep. The local social services team became involved after a neighbour's complaint, and contacted her GP for information. She had not seen her patient for over two years, so visited her at home. Mrs E. was very emotional, expressed many strange and unlikely ideas about her neighbours, and her home was disorganized and dirty, with little evidence of food in the kitchen. The GP asked for a formal mental health assessment, and the next day met two social workers at Mrs E.'s home. A sharp exchange followed about whether Mrs E. should be viewed as frail, vulnerable, and deluded (the doctor's view), or as eccentric, robust, but racist (the social workers' perception).

In 1984, Sheppard[53] looked at referrals to a mental health team from all sources and noticed that communication between GPs and social workers was infrequent, mostly taking place by telephone. This was markedly different to communication between community psychiatric nurses (CPNs) and GPs, which usually involved a letter from the CPN to the GP keeping them informed of progress in the case. Sheppard noted that compared to CPNs, social workers were clearly more reluctant to contact GPs and GPs were more reluctant to contact social workers. A community care development officer helped to facilitate the contract negotiations between social services in the Devon practice mentioned above.[51] She pointed out that the practice rarely communicated with the social services department by letter, their chosen communication method with all other agencies. The practice admitted that they had never considered this before.

We shall return to the relationships between social and primary care in more detail in Chapters 2 and 3, noting now that social care could not have been the salvation for innovative primary care for older people in the 1980s. First we must deal with the first attempt to create a national programme of primary care for older people through annual screening – the 75-and-over checks introduced in the 1990 general practitioner contract change. Stimulated by the research into assessment of older people in the community, this programme could have been an opportunity to test out assessment techniques, learn from the experiences of the previous decades, and absorb the sometimes negative lessons (for older people in the community) of closer collaboration with social care. As we shall see in Chapter 2, the opportunity was missed and the 'politics of the second best' reasserted itself. Secondly, we will review the changes that occurred in the social care of older people, and the legacy of problems that primary care groups must now manage.

References

1 Anderson WF & Cowan JR A consultative health centre for older people. *Lancet* 1955; 2:239–40.

2 Williamson J, Stokoe IH, Gray S, *et al.* Old people at home: their unreported needs *Lancet* 1964; 1:1117–20.

3 Klein R *The politics of the NHS.* Longman, London 1990.

4 Andrews K & Brocklehurst J *British geriatric medicine in the 1980s.* King Edward's Hospital Fund for London 1987.

5 Taylor RC & Buckley EG *Preventive care of the elderly: a review of current developments.* Royal College of General Practitioners, Occasional paper 35, London 1987.

6 Williams I A case for screening the elderly. *Update* 1975; 2:1275–85.

7 Tulloch AJ & Moore VL A randomised controlled trial of geriatric screening and surveillance in general practice. *BMJ* 1979; 29:733–42.

8 Williams I A follow-up of geriatric patients after socio-medical assessment. *Journal of the Royal College of General Practioners* 1974; **24**:341–6.

9 Ebrahim S, Hedley R, & Sheldon M Low levels of ill health among elderly non-consulters in general practice. *British Medical Journal* 1984; **289**:1273–5.

10 British Geriatrics Society & the Health Visitors Association *Health visiting for the health of the aged: a joint policy statement.* BGS/HVA, London 1986.

11 Butler MM Health visitors' use of risk criteria in an experimental screening project. In Taylor RC & Buckley EG (eds) *Preventive care of the elderly: a review of current developments.* Occasional paper 35. Royal College of General Practitioners, London 1987.

12 Macleod E & Mein P The nursing care team: a task force approach. In Taylor RC & Buckley EG (eds) *Preventive care of the elderly: a review of current developments.* Occasional Paper 35. Royal College of General Practitioners, London 1987.

13 Freer C Detecting hidden needs in the elderly: screening or case finding. In Taylor RC & Buckley EG (eds) *Preventive care of the elderly: a review of current developments.* Occasional Paper 35. Royal College of General Practitioners, London 1987.

14 Tulloch AJ Evaluation of geriatric screening: a review. In Taylor RC & Buckley EG (eds) *Preventive care of the elderly: a review of current developments.* Occasional Paper 35. Royal College of General Practitioners, London 1987.

15 Williams EI Scope for intervention following case identification. In Taylor RC & Buckley EG (eds) *Preventive care of the elderly: a review of current developments* Occasional Paper 35. Royal College of General Practitioners, London 1987.

16 Kewley J Self-help for the elderly. *Community View*, April 1984.

17 Drennan V Working with groups of elderly people. In Day L (eds) *Health visiting and older people.* Health Education Authority, London 1987.

18 Williams I *Caring for older people in the community.* Radcliffe, Oxford 1995.

19 Williams EI & Wallace P *Health checks for people aged 75 and over.* Occasional paper 59. Royal College of General Practitioners, London 1993.

20 Stuck AE, Siu AL, Wieland GD, *et al.* Effects of a comprehensive geriatric assessment on survival, residence and function: a meta-analysis of controlled trials. *Lancet* 1993; **342**:1032–6.

21 Wallace P The Paddington linkworker project. Personal communication.

22 Chung S Health visiting the elderly. *Nursing Mirror* 1985: **June 5th.**

23 Day L A health visitor's view of prevention. *Geriatric Medicine* 1983; **XIII**(9): 656–61.

24 Fitton JM Health visiting the elderly: nurse managers' views. *Nursing Times* 1984; **80**:59–61.

25 Luker KA Screening the well elderly in general practice. *Midwife, Health Visitor & Community Nurse* 1982; **18**(6):222–9.

26 Drennan V Developments in health visiting. *Health Visitor* 1986; **59**(4):108–10.

27 Drennan V   A feasibility study into the screening of elderly people in an inner city area. *While A Research in Preventive Community Nursing Care.* John Wiley, London 1986.

28 Luker K A Health visiting & the elderly. *Nursing Times Occasional Papers* 1981; **77**(35):137–40.

29 Phillipson C   Health visiting and older people: a review of current trends. *Health Visitor* 1985; **58**(12):357–8.

30 Ward RA. *The aging experience.*   Harper & Row, New York, 1984.

31 Victor CR   *Old age in modern society: a textbook of social gerontology.* Chapman & Hall, London 1989.

32 Blaxter M   *Health & lifestyles*, Routledge. London 1990.

33 Stainton-Rogers W *Explaining health and illness: an exploration of diversity* Harvester, Hemel Hempstead 1991.

34 Sidell M   *Health in old age: myth, mystery and management.* Open University Press Buckingham 1995.

35 Conway S & Hockey J   Resisting the 'mask' of old age?: the social meaning of lay health beliefs in later life. *Ageing & Society* 1998; **18**:469–94.

36 Williams RGA *The protestant legacy: attitudes to death and illness amongst older Aberdonians.* Oxford University Press, Oxford 1990.

37 Townsend P The structured dependency of the elderly. *Ageing & Society* 1981; **1**; 5–28.

38 Rowlings C   *Society work with older people.* Allen & Unwin, London 1987.

39 Chandler J   Attitudes of nursing personnel towards the elderly. *Gerontologist* 1986; **26**(4):551–5.

40 Luker K   Health visitor involvement with the elderly. In Taylor RC & Buckley EG *Preventive care of the elderly: a review of current developments* . Occassional Paper 35. Royal College of General Practitioners, London 1987.

41 Philipson C & Strang P   *Health education and older people : the role of paid carers* . Health Education Council /University of Keele, Keele 1984.

42 Biggs S Groupwork and professional attitudes to old age. In Morgan K (ed) *Gerontology: responding to an ageing society.* Jessica Kingsley, London 1992.

43 Biggs S Ageism and confronting ageing: experiential groupwork to examine attitudes to old age. *Journal of Social Work Practice* 1990; **4**:49–65.

44 Itzin K Ageism awareness and training. In Phillipson C, Bernard M & Strang P (eds) *Dependency and interdependency in old age.* Croom Helm, London 1986.

45 Antonovsky A   The sense of coherence as a determinant of health. In Matarazzo JP (ed) *Behaviour and health.* Wiley, New York 1984.

46 Levitt R *The Reorganized National Health Services.* Croom Helm, London 1976.

47 Davies B   Resources, needs and outcomes in community services – why academic caution is useful. In Morgan K (ed) *Gerontology: responding to an ageing society.* Jessica

Kingsley, London 1992.

48 Dickie S *Evaluation of the 75-and-over health checks: report 3 – the social services–primary care interface.* Department of Primary Care and Population Sciences, UCLMS 1996.

49 Dickie S & Iliffe S Bridging the gap between social services and primary care. *British Journal of Health Care Management* 1996; **2**(5):258–62.

50 Sheppard M Communications between general practitioners and a social services department. *British Journal of Social Work* 1985; **15**:15–47.

51 Morris R Community care and the fundholder. *British Medical Journal* 1993; **306**:635–7.

52 Huntingdon J *Social work and general practice: collaboration or conflict?* George Allen & Unwin, London 1991.

53 Sheppard M Contact and collaboration with general practitioners: a comparison of social workers and community psychiatric nurses. *British Journal of Social Work* 1992; **22**:419–36.

CHAPTER TWO

The 75-and-over screening programme and the Community Care act – one step forwards, two steps back?

In 1990 the government unilaterally changed the conditions of service for general practitioners, introducing a contractual obligation on members of primary health care teams to offer annual assessments of health to patients aged 75 and over.[1] These offers of assessment, which have to be made in writing, should be based on a home visit unless otherwise requested by the patient, and should include the following headings:

- *sensory function*
- *mobility*
- *mental condition*
- *physical condition, including continence*
- *social environment*
- *medication use.*

Whilst there had been extensive research into the possible benefits of regular screening or assessment of older people (see Chapter 1), at the time of the introduction of the 75-and-over checks there was still a lack of conclusive evidence that routine screening of whole populations was worthwhile. Nor was there a consensus on the best methods for such a screening approach, despite nearly 40 years of study.[2]

As suggested in the first chapter, many aspects of the elderly screening programme built into the new GP contract lacked a scientific basis. For example, information about the workload implications of the annual assessment package became available to general practitioners only after April 1990, suggesting that costing (let alone cost–benefit analysis) had not been performed in the contract's planning stages.[3, 4] Undoubtedly the lack of a plausible evidence base, and the lack of guidance on how to carry out the 75-and-over assessments, added to their unpopularity with GPs, who already resented the imposition of the 1990 contract upon them, and led to piecemeal and often unenthusiastic implementation of the programme.[5] Where assessment tasks

21

were undertaken at all they were delegated to practice nurses. and they have been given low priority by the local NHS administration[6] which (with a few exceptions) has neither provided leadership nor training for the programme, nor policed its implementation. In this chapter we will examine the need for an annual assessment of the 75-and-over age group, and redefine the term 'assessment' in more productive ways, before reviewing the other major change in services for older people, the NHS and Community Care Act.

Why 75?

Not only is the logic of whole-population screening questionable, but the choice of 75 (or any other age) for an assessment is arbitrary and may not be the most appropriate given the limited resources available in primary care. Vetter and colleagues have challenged the value of screening programmes beginning at 75, through re-analysis of data from an intervention trial using health visitors,[7] showing that some problems occur much earlier in life and should therefore be considered and addressed at a younger age. We want to explore the implications of this through the analysis of data from a random sample of patients over the age of 74 involved in a study covering all the elements of the annual assessment of the 75-and-over age group.

This will show that the older population is not homogenous, that annual screening may be too often for some and too infrequent for others, and that different assessment methods might be needed at different ages. It serves as an example of the information that can be gleaned from primary care research, even if it is not of an experimental kind.

Primary care research

General practitioners in nine practices in the London boroughs of Brent and Islington agreed to allow access to their age–sex registers, from which the names and addresses of all registered patients aged 75 and over were extracted. A random sample (239) were interviewed in depth, and represent the likely results from assessment of the patients of an 'average' two-doctor partnership. The methods used are described in detail in other reports from this two boroughs study.[3,4]

The general practice medical records of all elderly patients participating were scrutinized by an experienced nurse coordinating the fieldwork and all major diagnoses were recorded. All participants had a brief interview which included the Mini Mental State Examination, a measure of cognitive function that can serve as a pointer to dementia, if interpreted cautiously. Data were collected about the individual's actual and potential support network, mobility inside and outside the home, current medication, recent medical problems (including falls in the previous three months, experience of pain, and accidents, injuries, or chronic diseases that had impaired daily living in the previous year), hearing, vision, and urinary continence. The capacity to perform home tasks and tasks of personal care was assessed using a validated activities of daily living (ADL)

22

schedule. Prescribed medication used regularly was checked by the interviewer, and an assessment of mobility was also made. The results are therefore those that might be found from the application of the 75 -and-over screening assessment to the whole older population of a small general practice.

Social circumstances

The proportion of older people living alone did not increase significantly with age (Table 2.1). The majority received one or two social visits each month and this did not differ significantly between age groups. Children and neighbours were the main visitors, and visitors from voluntary organizations and church groups were uncommon. Most older people did not go out regularly (more

Table 2.1 *Social circumstances, support, mobility and personal and home care by age group*

	Age group		
	75–79 (n = 116) %	80–84 (n = 85) %	85+ (n = 38) %
SOCIAL CIRCUMSTANCES			
Lives alone	44	55	58
visitors	11	7	11
social outings	68	64	75
help in emergency	16	18	13
help at night	22	20	21
supportive relationship	14	12	18
MOBILITY			
Moderate or severe impairment	**14**	**27**	**45**
Up/down stairs unaided*	**96**	**86**	**74**
Mobile indoors unaided*	100	97	95
Mobile outdoors unaided*	**95**	**73**	**58**
Taking regular exercise	28	15	16
PERSONAL CARE			
Help needed with bathing	**11**	**22**	**47**
Problems with feet	39	45	34
HOME CARE			
Help needed with housework	14	33	40
Help needed with shopping	13	42	50
Help needed with meal preparation	10	14	32

* *Not requiring another person's assistance.*
Text and values in bold show statistically significant changes with advancing age.

than once a month) to a social or other kind of club. About 15% of each band said they had no one whom they could contact in an emergency and one in five in each age band had no source of help at night. Similar proportions in each band reported that they did not have anyone to whom they could talk about private matters, turn to in a crisis, or with whom they could feel at ease (Table 2.1). It is difficult to see why information about social contacts needs to be updated annually, rather than when change occurs.

Mobility

Self-reported mobility decreased significantly with age, as did the proportion of the study participants rated by an observer as having moderate to severe impairment of mobility (Table 2.1). More than one in 10 reported significant loss of mobility at 75 years, and arguably their disability should already be known to their GPs before that age. Physical activity promotion, as an antidote to functional loss, should begin at an earlier age. Although the only jogger encountered in this study was 80 years old, regular exercise was taken by only a quarter of those aged 75–79, and by significantly fewer amongst those aged 80 and over.

Home and personal care

The great majority of the youngest age group needed no help to perform such daily activities as housework, preparing food and drink, and shopping but these became significant problems in the older age groups (Table 2.1). There was a fivefold difference in the proportion needing help with bathing between the 75–79 and 85-and-over age bands. Needs assessment might be better aimed at the half of the 85-and-over age group who need help with bathing, and not at the near 90% of the 75–79 age group who do not. Problems with feet – bunions, corns, bent toes, or long toenails – sufficient to impair mobility were reported by over a third of each age band. Why should attempts to improve the feet of older people as a group wait until 75?

Sensory loss

Participants' responses to questions about vision and hearing are shown in Table 2.2. Inability to recognize a friend, even if using glasses, showed no statistically significant change with age, but the ability to read newspapers was significantly reduced amongst the very elderly. Amongst those with glasses the proportions in each age band unable to read a newspaper were: 75–79, 2%; 80–84, 8%; 85 and over, 22%. The proportion with substantially reduced hearing doubled between the younger and older age bands, as did the possession of hearing aids. These estimates of sensory loss are likely to under-report the scale of the problem because individuals adapt to slowly developing impairment and may not recognize its encroachment on their lives, but the lower prevalence of reduced visual or auditory function at younger ages suggests that this age group does not necessarily need the same assessment approach as their older peers

Table 2.2 *Hearing and vision loss, by age group*

	Age Group		
	75–79 (n=116) %	80–84 (n=85) %	85+ (n=38) %
SENSORY FUNCTIONS			
Wears glasses	92	91	82
Cannot recognize friend across road	**9**	**12**	**14**
Cannot recognize friend across room	2	2	8
Cannot read newspaper	3.5	10	19
Uses hearing aid	15	22	28
Cannot understand normal voice across room	19	15	31

Text and values in bold show statistically significant changes with advancing age.

Physical and mental health

Urinary incontinence occurred more frequently amongst women than men, and was not significantly more prevalent in the older age bands (Table 2.3), but its prevalence at 75 suggests that detection at an earlier age might be more appropriate. Persistent pain, experienced throughout or during most of the day, occurred in roughly the same proportions in each age band (Table 2.3). There were no statistically significant differences between the age bands in the proportions reporting impairment of daily life through chronic disease, accident, or injury in the past year, nor falls in the previous three months. However, falls appeared to become more serious in the older age bands; amongst the 75–79 age group 41% (n=11) were unable to get up unaided, but amongst those aged 85 and over the proportion was 71% (n=5). The proportions of people describing their health as worse than that of their peers remained similar in all three age bands. (Table 2.3). There were no significant differences between the age bands in the proportions taking two or more prescribed medicines regularly, nor in the proportions with two or more diagnoses recorded in their GPs notes.

Possible cases of depression and dementia aggregated to make a category of 'significant psychiatric disorder' showed no statistically significant difference in prevalence between age bands, although this hides the increase in dementia

Table 2.3 *Incontinence, medication use, and mental and physical health, by age group*

	Age group		
	75–79 (n=116) %	80–84 (n=85) %	85+ (n=38) %
URINARY INCONTINENCE			
Men	5	14	18
Women	32	26	8
USE OF PRESCRIBED MEDICATION			
No medicine	39	25	34
One medicine	16	26	17
Two or more medicines	46	49	49
MENTAL HEALTH			
Major psychiatric disorder	26	38	43
Life satisfaction poor	**4**	**10**	**21**
PHYSICAL HEALTH			
Perceived poor health	4	6	3
Persistent pain	46	26	24
Chronic disease or injury	38	39	45
Recent fall	22	26	18
No diagnoses	20	21	19
Two or more diagnoses	34	33	51

Text and values in bold show statistically significant changes with advancing age.

to over 20% in the 85-and-over age group, and the reduction in the prevalence of depression symptoms with advancing age. Satisfaction with life, taking into consideration any current problems, was rated as poor by significantly more individuals in the older age bands (Table 2.3). What then is the rationale for routinely assessing older people between the ages of 75 and 79 for dementia, when it is uncommon, but not having a more intense focus on the very old, whose falls become increasingly serious with advancing age?

This study, conducted in general practice by GPs and nurses, relies more on self-reported impairment than on observation, and contains no element of examination other than use of validated psychiatric rating scales. It may, therefore, under- or overstate the extent of impairment. However, there are three reasons for using self-report as the basis for assessment of the health of older people. Firstly, perceived health status amongst older people has been found to accord well with objective health status.[8] Taylor and Ford's study in Aberdeen also suggested that stoical tolerance of illness or impairment was less prevalent than had been previously thought.[9] Secondly, self-reported impairment amongst older people in the community is a good predictor of future service use.[10] Finally, use of a self-completed questionnaire has been shown to be an effective first step in identifying older people needing further assessment.[11, 12, 13]

The population studied is small enough for small but important differences to be missed, especially when analysing data from the most elderly age band – those aged 85 and over – and therefore the results need cautious interpretation. Because the study is cross-sectional it is not possible to distinguish ageing effects from cohort differences, making generalization to future populations of older people speculative. Nevertheless, these findings represent the possible yield from a comprehensive mass screening of a predominantly white, working-class, elderly population, using self-report as the main source of data.

Several characteristics were similarly prevalent in all three age bands, including social circumstances, regular use of prescribed medication, and number of diagnoses recorded in the general practice record. It is difficult to see why social circumstances need to be reviewed annually, rather than when they change, especially since for this population lone status was not associated with higher morbidity [14] and lack of confiding relationships was not associated with depression.[15] Medication review is an important task, given the extent of iatrogenesis.[16] but annual assessment seems arbitrary and more frequent review may be appropriate, and should anyway be a routine component of the case management approach that we will describe later. One in five of each band had no significant diagnoses recorded in the general practice record, and an even larger proportion had no regular medication prescribed. Poor-quality recording may account for some of this apparently healthy group, but GPs are rarely criticized for prescribing too little for their elderly patients, and the fact that between a quarter and a third of each age band were not receiving repeat medicines suggests that a significant minority of the very elderly remain relatively well.

This does not mean that they lacked potentially remediable impairments, and we do not want to promote a nihilistic approach to anticipatory care for older people. There is much that can be done, but it needs to be tailored to individuals, problems, and advancing age, not straitjacketed into a simplistic assessment system. The prevalence of hearing and visual loss amongst the 75–79 age group was high, and the well-documented association between both hearing and vision loss and falls,[17] together with the morbidity and mortality associated with falls,[18] makes assessment of these senses an important task. In the 85-and-over age band five times as many people could not read the newspaper, even when wearing glasses, than amongst those aged 75–79. This may reflect not only untreatable macular degeneration but also undetected and potentially treatable glaucoma, cataract, and retinopathy. Annual assessment of vision may well be appropriate for the older age bands, although it is arguable that it should be done by optometrists rather than general practitioners, given the apparent tendency to delay referral and the problematic lack of accuracy in identifying retinopathy, even after training.[19] Hearing loss may similarly deserve regular assessment, both for those with hearing aids whose impairment cannot be assumed to be reduced and amongst those without aids. Although screening for hearing loss could usefully begin at a much earlier age[20] there remains considerable scope for ameliorating deafness in the elderly. [21]

Urinary incontinence has a deleterious effect on quality of life,[22] may be an important factor in institutionalizing elderly people,[23] and is expensive for health services. Intervention can improve the quality of life in a proportion of people suffering with urinary incontinence.[24] Urinary incontinence was prevalent in all age bands, but was not significantly more prevalent amongst those aged 80 and over, supporting Jolleys' findings from a study in one practice.[25] Nearly a third of women in the 75–79 age band reported at least occasional urinary incontinence, suggesting that screening at 75 may be unnecessarily late. Amongst the 85-and-over age band a higher proportion of men than women reported urinary incontinence, possibly reflecting the increased prevalence of advanced prostatism. Responses to the hidden problem of incontinence will be discussed further in Chapter 8.

Impairment of mobility and with personal and home care tasks was significantly higher in the older age bands, reflecting the known rising prevalence of disability with age,[26] but as reported elsewhere almost all of those needing support services were in contact with them at the time of the study, and few requested extra help[4, 5]. The rationale for annual assessment of impairment in addition to ongoing clinical review and case management is difficult to see, but if such assessment is justified probably it should be concentrated on the older age bands where reported impairment is greatest.

General practitioners are rightly critical of the contractual obligation to offer annual assessments to the 75-and-over age group. A significant minority do not honour this obligation and anecdotal evidence suggests that many others fail to be systematic and comprehensive. The danger in this situation is that assessment of the elderly may be discredited because of the imposition of an unfocused screening programme that underemphasizes the need for proper case management. Primary care professionals cannot abandon elderly people with significant medical problems or impairments, but may be better employed in case-finding, developing a database for the elderly population of the practice, auditing the quality of care, and developing teamwork skills. Assessment of the health of older people is necessary, but not necessarily in the form of screening of whole populations. Another approach is needed involving a different use of the 'term assessment'. We need to step back from the prescriptiveness of the 1990 contract and think about what is being assessed, why and for whom.

From screening to assessment

The fundamental questions about the uses of assessment of older people which had been debated before 1990 were not answered by the introduction of the 75-and-over screening programme. From that debate we can summarize the purposes of assessment in older age groups in five ways:

(1) preventive screening that aims to avoid future problems through identification of risk factors amenable to intervention, or through earlier diagnosis of pathology where earlier intervention can reduce morbidity or disability; early identification of problems means that primary care for older people is concerned not just with intervention but also with providing the signposts to other types of services and support networks
(2) measuring the severity of diseases or disabilities in individuals and monitoring their progress during treatment or therapy
(3) auditing the quality and effectiveness of clinical work, whether therapeutic or remedial
(4) creating a database for rational resource allocation by measuring the scale of any set of problems and attempting to predict future trends
(5) and basic research requiring population and cohort studies where not enough is yet known about the size, distribution, and correlates of any significant problem.

As we have shown, in the early 1990s preventive screening of older populations could not be supported by the available evidence. Screening in any form is of little value if little is done about the problems identified. For example, we know that descriptive studies show that screening yields significant amounts of unmet need, but also that patients and professionals alike do not necessarily do anything about some needs identified this way.[27] There are also hints that some unmet need may remain unmet for complex reasons as much to do with the individual's frame of mind and expectations as with the alertness or sensitivity of services.[28]

Similarly, whilst RCTs performed up to 1990 had shown that screening and intervention could reduce mortality and in-patient stay, and increase referral rates and patient satisfaction, there have been no studies to measure the effects of these changes on either the health service or the private economy of individuals and families. Nor have there been any studies of how useful patients and their families or neighbours actually found the assessments they received, even though the support for some form of regular 'check' is widespread amongst older people themselves and their families. We are left, then, with the other senses of the word 'assessment', none of which require whole-population screening, and all of which are compatible with carefully organized, systematic health care. If annual assessments for all those aged 75 or more make little sense, and any form of population screening is suspect, what needs to change in primary care practice? And what should practitioners do with the 75-and-over checks, which remain a contractual obligation? We will answer these questions in Chapter 3, after discussing the popularity of the 75-and-over checks with older people in the light of their satisfaction with general practice.

The older consumer

Overall satisfaction with GP services is high amongst the older population, but decreases as questions about the quality of care become more specific.[29] The generation born around the time of the First World War may be reluctant to bother the doctor, take the view that they need to use medical care sparingly, and feel ill-equipped to challenge medical perceptions, but they do have specific criticisms that are carefully guarded from superficial enquiry. GPs are seen as being unwilling to visit, sometimes insensitive, and unlikely to give enough information.[30]

> Mrs F.'s daughter asked for a home visit late one Friday afternoon because her mother had taken to her bed and stopped eating. Her GP duly but reluctantly visited this 86-year-old, whose main medical problem was recurrent urinary tract infection, plodding up seven floors of the tower block where she lived because the lifts were out of order. Mrs F. was in bed, grumbling, but seemed pleased to see her usual doctor. 'That young doctor that came round the other day didn't stay a minute,' she complained, 'and she just prodded my stomach. She didn't even take my pulse,' she added as her GP took her pulse. When finally told that she had another bladder infection she said she had guessed as much, and would have taken the medicine left by the previous doctor (amoxicillin) if she had known what it was for.

Unwillingness to visit as a criticism may surprise GPs whose home visits are likely to focus on their older patients, but the number of visits has decreased across all age groups, and the 'social visit' so popular as reassurance that someone cares is unlikely to be as commonplace as it was a generation ago. Insensitivity might also strike a cohort of doctors better trained in communication skills than their predecessors as an unjust criticism, but whilst the professional moves on from each consultation to the rest of a busy day, the patient is left to mull over every word. Too hearty an approach to prostate symptoms or arthritic joints, and too ready an attribution of ailments to ageing, may be remembered when other, more accurate and appropriate perceptions are not.

The pattern of deferential social distance between older patient and doctor, and reluctance to ask questions, report failure to improve, describe adverse effects, or challenge therapies, is changing. A decade or more of government-sponsored medical consumerism has had an effect on older people and their families, and every clinician has encountered the demand that 'something must be done' for older patients, even if this seems unrealistic and irrational to the professional. Medical consumerism, in the form of buyers' challenges to sellers' claims, replaces faith and trust with doubt and caution and appears to be a universal phenomenon, in developed and developing countries alike.[31] However, consumerist attitudes are more common than consumerist behaviour, with attitudes being expressed in changed behaviour only after people become ill and experience the apparent failure of medical treatments. Typically, the burden of chronic disease that cannot be relieved by current therapies triggers changes in the perceptions patients hold of their doctors and nurses. Naïve trust in professional potency gives way to disenchantment with medicine as failure occurs, which is in turn replaced by a tactic of guarded alliance.[32] Guarded alliances may take different forms, including hero worship, resignation, or consumerism of the type discussed above.

Mr A.'s depression lifted, and he remained as active as his impairment allowed, even trying an aerobics class at the local leisure centre for a while. But he never lost the uncomfortable feelings in the arm affected by the stroke, and this distressed him. He visited his GP every month to have his blood pressure checked and almost always asked what more could be done about his arm symptoms. Although his doctor never had any new ideas, Mr A. always left the consultation saying that only his doctor kept him alive and active.

Mrs B.'s grief at her husband's death waxed and waned for much longer than her GP expected. She became very tired, but her doctor could not find any explanation for this other than her bereavement. She began to look for solutions to her tiredness from many different sources, including the cardiology ward in the hospital where her husband had been treated, the local health food shop, and a private naturopath. She would bring clippings from newspapers and magazines, and packets of remedies that friends had bought and lent to her, for her doctor to see and comment upon. She always asked whether her lassitude was really due to her bereavement, but in a way that made her own scepticism clear.

GPs and other primary care professionals may want to promote the team-playing (or producerism) in which the patient becomes a co-worker in maintaining or promoting health. To do this we will have to address the issues about contact, communication, and information exchange that emerge in critical accounts of primary care services. Decisions about what to do about health and illness depend on relevant knowledge, which younger professionals may assume older people have acquired experientially, over time. This assumption may be unfounded in cohorts where formal education after 14 or 16 years was uncommon, and may be confounded by the passive, withdrawn state adopted by some people as they age (see Chapter 1). Those working with an older population need to think about the five types of knowledge needed for self-care:[33]

(1) diagnostic skills, such as taking a temperature, measuring the pulse, or doing breast self examination
(2) treatment skills for common, acute, and self-limiting illness or injuries
(3) chronic illness management, including self-monitoring and concordance with medication
(4) health promotion, including physical activity and healthy eating
(5) routes to help, including reliable knowledge as well as professional help.

This list of knowledge types looks short but each heading subsumes huge amounts of information. How can any attempt to address this educational agenda be carried out in practice without patronizing or infantilizing older patients? Is such an approach compatible with current knowledge about the impact of interventions and with current resources , and is it ethical to impose an agenda of self-reliance on patients whose perceptions of need and support may be much different and much simpler?

At 80, Mrs G. had near perfect recall of the plots of all of Shakespeare's plays, could discuss the merits of new and old productions on stage and television, and had strong views on the Bard's contemporaries and rivals. Although she had left school at 16, much later than most of her contemporaries, she had worked as a clerk, barmaid, or shop assistant all her life, where she amazed her fellow workers with her erudition. But when it came to her health she ran out of words, telephoning her family to enquire about the significance and treatment of everyday symptoms that she had encountered many times before. Responding to an invitation to a 75-and -over check, she told the practice nurse that her left leg hurt, but omitted to say that she drank enough sherry at lunchtime to make her sleep all afternoon. Discussing the long-standing and increasingly disabling limb pain with her family, she described the nurse as 'kind' but was unable to recall any specific advice given and did not feel that her leg pain warranted further investigation – a feeling that the nurse agreed with.

The ethics of assessment

To be ethically acceptable, assessment of elderly people should be acceptable to the people themselves, have a validated process with sensitive and specific instruments, and identify remediable problems for which resources exist. The assessment process should yield more benefits than dangers – particularly avoiding the medicalization of old age, over-treatment, and poor-quality superficial judgements that verge on saying 'it's your age' – whilst preserving confidentiality. Annual screening of the kind required by the current GP contract does not fulfil these criteria, and logically should not be pursued in its present form, even though the evidence in favour of highly selective interventions for some older people with disabilities is now growing, mostly from work carried out in North America and Europe. The arguments for a limited assessment package with very specific content to replace the 75-and-over checks are reviewed in the next chapter, but here we are concerned with the overall approach to the health of older people that could and should be taken in primary care. Is the new American-style comprehensive geriatric assessment that approach?

Comprehensive geriatric assessment and systematic case management

The prevention or amelioration of established disease or disability through comprehensive geriatric assessment (CGA) has been shown to be effective in some populations. The likelihood that an older individual will be living at home with better functional ability one year after CGA doubles compared with 'normal care' controls.[34] Similarly, older patients with cardiac failure benefit from intensive home-based review with improved functional status, less frequent hospital admission, and reduced length of in-patient stay.[35] The critical factor appears to be systematic management of problems that are identified.

However, these are examples of tertiary prevention in older adults with existing symptomatic disease who are at high risk of becoming further disabled, not primary prevention as apparently envisaged in the 75-and-over screening programme. Whilst some research published since 1990 does suggest that primary and secondary prevention is possible, it is limited. Annual comprehensive geriatric assessment followed by periodic in-home nurse practitioner review did reduce nursing home admissions and did slow functional decline in a non-disabled American population.[36] Similarly, modifying a set of predisposing factors for falls and incontinence may prevent or delay the onset of functional dependence.[37]

These may be important signs that targeted primary and secondary preventive interventions are worthwhile in the community, but they do not yet add up to conclusive evidence and do not provide a retrospective justification for the approach taken in British general practice in 1990. They are based on work in a different health care system, and are the types of research project where the results are diluted once they are applied to real-world community programmes, largely because relatively small changes in the intervention may reduce its effectiveness. Primary and secondary prevention of most morbidity and disability in the older population awaits identification of critical risk factors for disability, clarification of the causal mechanisms promoting disability, clear understanding of which components of any intervention are effective, and delineation of the interplay between functional decline and disability, over time.[38] Primary care workers may have much to contribute to these tasks in the course of their own research and development efforts, but their clinical work will need a different approach to assessment if it is to be fruitful and sustainable (Box 2.1).

In summary, the form of assessment with the fewest ethical objections, most relevant to individuals, and closest to usual practice is comprehensive and systematic case management with a proactive dimension of case-finding, representing the second and third meanings given above. This approach will be discussed in more detail in the next chapter, after we have returned to the relationship between general practice and social services because assessment of health that does not measure social needs in older people can be neither comprehensive nor systematic.

Social care for older people in the 1980s

By the 1980s the failure to extend social services provision in response to rising need (created largely by demographic change) had resulted in a growing 'care gap' between the need for care and the provision of domiciliary services.[39]

Box 2.1 *A research agenda for primary care*

The research networks now growing in primary care could answer many questions of relevance to disability and the health of older people:

- What are the risk factors for disability?
- How do they operate, and why do they affect some but not others?
- What interventions are possible, and how acceptable and effective are they?
- What is the natural history of functional decline?

The amount of care provided by family, friends, and neighbours (so-called informal carers) increased whilst institutional budgets continued to dominate both health and social services.[40] Urgent economic pressures in the late seventies plus a new orientation in government attitude produced a change in policy towards social care. The emphasis was shifted away from care *in* the community, supported by local authority personnel, towards a confusing mixture of care *by* the community itself and private care, regardless of whether in domiciliary or institutional settings. The protected status of personal social services (PSS) spending was ended, and the coordination and monitoring of local service provision was abandoned and replaced by an increasing reliance on non-statutory forms of welfare.[41]

The private sector for provision of care to older people was promoted by reducing the resources available to local authorities and using rate-capping to enforce the new policy.[42] The 1980s witnessed the fastest rate of growth in residential and nursing home places of this century, and the social security budget fuelling this increase became the fastest growing item of public expenditure, from £10 million in 1979 to well over £2 billion in 1995.

The government attempted to reduce the social services to residual organizations which provided those services which noone else could or would take on. Their function was seen as one of being a long-stop for the very special needs going beyond the range of voluntary services, so that care in the community increasingly meant care *by* the community, in which the main role for the PSS was to backup and develop the assistance which is given by private and voluntary support.

The result was a social security budget which spiralled out of control and perverse incentives for older people requiring care to enter residential homes, despite the proclaimed policy of community care. Government attention in the early 1990s was focused almost exclusively on the organization of community care and the creation of an internal market utilizing a purchaser/provider split model familiar to those working in the NHS. The promises of real community care and an increased influence over care decisions were still made, with practical support for informal carers so that service users would be given *'a greater individual say in how they live their lives and the services they need to help them to do so'*.[43]

The perverse incentive has resulted in the oversupply of residential care places and tighter rationing of home-based care. Over the decade 1979–1989 the numbers of beds in the private residential sector trebled, to 31.1 places per 1000 people over 65. Yet it is estimated that only 11 places per 1000 people over the age of 65 are required to support severely disabled older people. A significant proportion of older people in private residential homes, perhaps as much as one-half, do not need to occupy residential places on the basis of disability. Substantial numbers are still entering residential homes because there is no reliable community-based alternative, where they encounter the dependency-creating aspects of residential regimes much earlier than they need.[43] This rapid expansion of the private sector has been biased towards the younger old, amongst whom need is less extensive than among the very elderly. For instance, between 1979 and 1989 there was a 38% growth in the numbers aged 85 and over and this was accompanied by a 12% rise in the number of private residential beds; yet while the population aged 65–74 declined by 9% there was a 15% growth in private provision for this group. The uncontrolled expansion of the private nursing and residential home sector militated against the distribution of services for frail older people according to need. To this inequity we must add the geographical maldistribution of residential and nursing homes, which have developed disproportionately in affluent areas at the expense of inner-city and peripheral populations. If the growing corporate involvement in nursing and residential home development fails to identify under-served areas as potential untapped niche markets, or if the whole market stagnates, geographical inequalities will persist.[44]

Some argue that the growth of the private sector of residential care is beneficial because it increases choice in a 'mixed economy of welfare'.[45] However, one result of the government's residualization strategy has been to cut local authority residential places for all age groups of older people, especially those aged 85 and over, whilst the building of sheltered housing for older people has fallen sharply. Yet genuine choice requires a range of alternative forms of care: public-sector homes, day care, the opportunity to remain in an ordinary dwelling with community support. Ironically, this sort of choice has been severely restricted by the 'perverse incentive' for older people to enter residential care created by social security payments.[46]

When it comes to entering a residential home the concept of 'choice' is rarely appropriate. The need for residential care usually arises because of a crisis of care in the informal sector, leaving little time to 'shop around' for alternatives, so that the promise of choice is often illusory.[47] The creation of a large private residential care sector has not resulted in greater choice for older people and their families. In one study in the late 1980s only a quarter of nursing home residents exercised any choice about the home they were admitted to, while nearly a quarter said that their admission resulted from unsolicited arrangements by a third party.[47]

Choice between private homes is restricted by factors such as geographical location (see above), waiting lists, and ability to pay, and homes may be bought and sold without reference to the residents, whilst the character of the home as well as an individual's living arrangements may be altered without consultation. The fees of some homes, coupled with the enforcement of the more stringent means test, has forced relatives and older people themselves to contribute towards the cost of long-term care. There are now numerous examples of people selling their homes to finance residential care. This policy development, which was never presented openly in any election manifesto, has enormous implications for relationships within families.

Health and social care in the 1990s

The NHS and Community Care Act 1990 was created out of three different policy agendas for long-term care of the elderly present since the 1950s. These were (i) to contain spending on health and social care; (ii) to promote the ethos of care provision in the community; and (iii) to improve collaboration between health and social care. It provided an opportunity to improve communications between primary and social care, but it also created so many problems for those caring for older people that the opportunity may have been lost. The question for GPs and community nurses, and in particular for the new primary care groups (PCGs) and trusts, is whether the negative effects of the Community Care Act can be overcome and the collaborative opportunities regained.

From April 1993, local authorities were given responsibility for assessment and then provision of an individual's welfare needs, based on the policy of the 1988 Griffiths Report.[48] Griffiths charged social services to:

'Identify and assess individuals' needs, taking full account of personal preferences (and those of informal carers) and design packages of care best suited to enabling the consumer to live as normal a life as possible.'

The aim of the Act was to encourage the provision of services so that people who would previously have been institutionalized could remain in the community. A fair test of this policy would be whether it reduced the proportion of social services spending on residential care in favour of community-based services, without worsening outcomes for those in need, loss of equity in provision of care, and decreased efficiency in service organization. As we shall see, the exact opposite has occurred, with major implications for older people, their families, and local services.

One such implication has been that services have been withdrawn from individuals with low levels of need and redirected towards those with higher levels of need, in an attempt to avert institutional care. As Davies has demonstrated very clearly,[49] this approach will not work because:

- those at high need of home support may not be at high risk of admission to a nursing or residential home
- half of those who do enter institutional care have no prior contact with community services
- removal of low levels of support may change the status of the patient, moving them into a higher risk category
- increased input of services to individuals with high needs who do seem to be at risk of admission to residential care may not have much impact on their disabilities and illnesses and on the pathway of subsequent care.

It seems that the same lack of critical thinking occurred in planning changes in social care as happened with the introduction of the 75-and-over assessments in general practice.

The largest group of people affected by the Griffiths reform of social care were the old. Those who would once have been cared for in long-stay NHS beds, under consultant care, were now more likely to remain at home where the responsibility for their health care fell on GPs and district nurses. If the Community Care Act's principle of home-based support were driving change we would expect collaboration between health and social care to move up the local policy agenda, with closer working between primary care and social services departments. While there is evidence that this happened between the local authorities and community health services, we shall demonstrate how this has not happened between local authorities and general practice .

The Act created a new distinction between 'health' – and thus financial responsibility of the health service – and 'social' care – the financial responsibility of the local authority. Most significant in trying to reach clarity on these terms was that 'social care' would be means tested and 'health care' free at the point of access. Social care was now defined to include all aspects of personal care and domestic tasks necessary for all aspects of daily living.[50] The previous decade's fighting over who should help old people wash and bath seemed to have ended in a negotiated truce, at least in terms of financial responsibility. The incremental moves by local authorities during the eighties to develop their home help services which provided personal care now became wholesale developments. Whether maintenance of personal hygiene and management of incontinence is funded by the health or local authority has not been agreed consistently across the country, and is rarely made explicit for the older person who may be financially assessed for these services dependent on local – usually verbal – agreements between agencies.

At the same time, the NHS and Community Care Act legislated for the local authorities and health authorities to introduce separate purchasing and providing functions, which fundamentally changed a number of roles and relationships , not least the conversion of the social worker into the care manager. The drive to use financial resources most effectively meant that both authorities had to develop 'mixed economies' of providers. While initially offering opportunities of greater integration for the person receiving care, the net effect has been to fragment the provision of care to older peoples in their homes between state 'not for profit' agencies and the commercial sector.

The responsibility to inform GPs of changing referral procedures for community care assessment fell on social services departments. However, GPs are not always an easy group to inform. The Nuffield Institute for Health studied six localities in 1992 to see what steps they were taking to involve GPs in the implementation of community care.[51] It found that in all areas social services were working closely with family health services authorities (FHSAs) to develop assessment arrangements that were acceptable to GPs, but were encountering problems. In one area joint conferences had to be repeatedly cancelled because of lack of response from GPs. In another, an initiative to develop a common assessment process, combining the social assessment with the GPs' 75-and-over check, was met with resistance in the pilot practices apparently because the GPs had developed their own 75-and-over assessment tool and saw no benefit in adopting a new one.

The British Medical Association (BMA) surveyed GPs, psychiatrists, geriatricians, and public health physicians before and after April 1993 about the implementation of the Act.[52] Over three-quarters of GPs did not recall being consulted by their local social services department before April 1993 and most were unaware of the changes. In the second survey in 1993, 36% of GPs and community specialists thought services had got worse while 40% thought consultation and joint training with social services had been poor. Only 10% thought there had been any improvement in communication.

A study conducted by a joint social service and primary care team in North Thames region investigated four areas, two suburban and two inner-city. A sample of GPs and social workers were interviewed six months before the implementation of the Community Care Act and subsequently. Six months before the reforms 37% of GPs contacted thought their relationship with social services was 'good or fairly good'. Almost a quarter of the GPs questioned six months and one year after the reforms thought that communication had deteriorated, while only 20% thought it had improved. Commonly cited difficulties on each side were problems making contact, a lack of face-to-face contact, and a lack of continuity in GPs' links with social services.[53]

Since the poor relationship between GPs and social workers stems in part from a lack of understanding of the differences in their working practices (see Chapter 1), interprofessional education may be one way of improving relationships. This is not a new idea. In the 1970s the Royal College of General Practitioners and the British Association of Social Workers formed a Standing Liaison Committee to promote collaboration in the training of GPs and social workers, and there are examples in the literature of joint facilitated groups for trainees from the two disciplines, where cases could be discussed from the two different perspectives.[54] Examples of current similar schemes are hard to find in the literature, but the issues around joint working will be reviewed in Chapter 4 on teamwork and in Chapter 12 on commissioning.

Levels of joint working range from attempts to evolve some kind of agreed understanding of each other's roles in the assessment process in community care,[44] for example by negotiating GP practice–social service department contracts, to various levels of social worker attachment to practices. Social worker attachments to practices were common in the 1970s, but became much more infrequent as local authorities had to cap spending in the 1980s. Half of all social services departments reported GP attachment of social workers in 1976, compared with 13.5% in 1991,[55] although practice attachment or some form of co-location of social and primary health care has begun to develop again since 1993. In the 1970s social workers were more likely to be 'generic' (generalist) and therefore a practice-based social worker would deal with many different types of case. As social service departments are now divided into specialist teams, whose remit varies from area to area, the 'generic' social worker who works in a practice now will only deal with adults with physical health problems, the majority of whom will be elderly. In theory this should allow better provision and coordination of medical and social care for older people. In reality the consequences of changes in social care have militated against such progress, in ways that every GP and community nurse has encountered, and with which every primary care group must now grapple .

The current state of community care

Tighter rationing of community care budgets means that in many places social care at home is available only to those who meet strict eligibility criteria, including financial. For this group, care is only provided up to a set financial ceiling and then institutional care becomes the only option. Frail older people who in previous decades, would have expected to receive some assistance are now being denied it. Instead family, friends and neighbours are being expected to provide care that was once the responsibility of the statutory authorities. Despite rhetoric about the new role of the social services consumer and listening to the views of carers, the majority of older people needing care, particularly those being discharged from hospital, do not have much choice in what they get. Social service care managers have been put in an impossible position of being expected to respond to the views of service users whilst keeping within budgets that are declining relative to the growth in need created by population ageing. What was trumpeted as a new needs-led service has quickly reverted to one which attempts to meet needs within tightly controlled and inadequate budgets. Not surprisingly, resources are being focused only on those with the most pressing needs and, as a consequence, the possibility of preventive and rehabilitative work is being reduced. The choice of remaining at home with support is only permitted within fixed financial per capita limits. Members of the boards of PCGs and trusts should note this experience.

The assessment system used in social care is compromised because, unlike its medical role model (more in geriatric medicine than in primary care), there is no guarantee of a service response. Social service care managers are placed in an invidious position because they cannot assess need if they are unable to meet that need, without the risk of legal action initiated by the person they have assessed, or by the family. In these circumstances it is virtually impossible for managers to be honest with service users and their carers.

For those frail and vulnerable people who are in limbo between the NHS and social services or those carers, often old and frail themselves, who are being driven to the end of their endurance by the need to provide 24–hour care to a spouse or parent suffering from depression, confusion, or dementia, community care can be a personal nightmare.

Deficiencies in community care policy

Over the last 50 years, the proportion of people aged 65 and over resident in homes or long-stay hospitals has actually increased, with a very marked increase in the eighties and nineties. The failure to develop effective community care has a long history, but there a number of lessons for primary care workers.

The first obstacle to effective community care of older people is the 'floodgates' mentality, which argues that if a high-quality community care service is provided, families will leave everything to the state and spending will go out of control. This fear is common currency amongst policy makers, yet there is no scientific evidence to sustain it. On the contrary, families remain the front-line providers of care regardless of what support is available externally, reflecting the complex process of decision-making within families concerning the care of older relatives, with social services being regarded as the last, not the first, resort.[56] The 'floodgates' argument reveals ignorance of the sociology of family relationships and the extent of reciprocity between the generations.

However, the nature of both the caring relationship and the family itself are changing rapidly. As a result of increased longevity families are having to care over longer and longer periods, but the ability (not the willingness) of kin to provide such care is being constrained by socio-demographic changes such as the reduction in family size, the ageing of spouse carers, the increase in female labour-force participation, and the rise in the divorce rate. Therefore families require more support, not less, if they are to sustain their caring relationships.

Unfortunately, fears about opening the floodgates have confined community care to a very limited back-stop or casualty service. This has had several negative consequences. It has weighed particularly heavily on women, who are more likely than men to provide personal and domestic care, and reinforced gender-based inequalities in the distribution of informal care. It has prevented the practice of community care from realizing its full potential with regard to prevention and rehabilitation. This approach to community care has placed too much responsibility on family carers and may well have increased the likelihood that caring relationships will break down.

European comparisons demonstrate the potential for a more effective partnership between the family and the state in the care of older people. Denmark has the most developed home care provision in the European Community with three times as many home carers as in Britain, so that in Denmark more than two-thirds of older people receiving care are getting help from the social services compared with only a quarter in the UK, whilst just over two-fifths of Danish older people are being helped by their families compared with three-fifths in the UK.[57] Denmark's superior community care provision has not resulted in a reduction in family care because community care is viewed in part as a mechanism to support the economic independence of women. Comparisons of family contact show similar patterns between the two countries, suggesting that community care does not result in the desertion of older people by their families.[58] Table 2.4 shows the extent and intensity (hours of support per week) of home-help provision for people aged 65 or more in the Nordic countries compared with all social care support for the same population in Britain in 1998.[59]

The concept of community care that has been pursued in the last 50 years is a very limited one amounting, at best, to a few hours home help support *in* the community. The potential for community care to operate in partnership with families to support their caring activities has not been allowed to develop, and the exclusion of health and housing from the narrow social services definition of community care has resulted in repeatedly unsuccessful attempts to improve coordination (see above). The need for active community support and community development has never been part of the approach to commu-

Table 2.4 *International comparison of social care provision*

Country	Cover (proportion 65 & over receiving support)	Intensity (hours per week)
Denmark	20	4.9
Finland	10	3.4
Norway	14	3.3
Sweden	14	6.8
England & Wales	4.6	3.2

nity care, although PCGs may be in a position to change this. Nor has the connection between economic policy and community care been on the agenda of service development, although that too is changing with the current focus on social exclusion as a major problem for society. The extent to which care *by* the community depends on care *for* the community has not been recognized.

Community care policy and practice have exhibited discriminatory attitudes towards older people, with a ready acceptance of institutional care as appropriate for older people when it was rejected long ago for children. The unified social service departments established following the Seebohm Report of 1968 were soon preoccupied with child care issues, a bias that was reinforced by each of the long series of inquiries into the death of children and the resulting statutory guidance or legislation. Social services departments function according to a client group hierarchy, with older people at the bottom,[60] so that social work with older people has been regarded as routine and low priority, just as it has in health visiting (see Chapter 1).

The continuation of these attitudes has been shown in work demonstrating that the service principles applied to people with learning difficulties, such as normalization and the right to an ordinary life, are overturned with regard to older people with learning difficulties in favour of the assumption of a service continuum from day care to domiciliary care to residential care. The quality of life of a person with learning difficulties and the support they may expect from the social services depends critically on their age.[61]

Primary care groups are inheriting a poisoned chalice of damaging policy and uneven practice when addressing the health and social care needs of an ageing population. The attempt to embed anticipatory care for older people into general practice has failed, for reasons that were predictable at the time of its introduction, and PCGs will need to reflect on alternative approaches without rushing into change. Changes in social care have been introduced on the basis of flimsy evidence of effectiveness and the opportunities for closer collaboration between primary care and social services have been undervalued or ignored. PCGs may not be able to alter the resources available to social care, at least in the short term, but they can work on the issues of collaboration and teamwork across disciplines. The agenda for PCGs is a large one, encompassing:

- the historical split between health and social care
- the change in the role of social worker to care manager
- the withdrawal of services from 'low dependency' individuals
- the introduction in social care of eligibility criteria and financial ceilings on provision
- the promotion of a mixed economy of provision whilst NHS provision of continuing-care beds has decreased
- the engagement of community health staff in joint working, with the exception of general practitioners.

We will develop some arguments about how these issues might be approached in outline in Chapter 3, and use the rest of this book to address them in more detail.

References

1 Department of Health *A new contract for general practice.* HMSO, London 1990.

2 Harris A Health checks for the over-75s: the doubt persists. *British Medical Journal* 1992; **305**: 599–600.

3 Iliffe S, Gallivan S, Haines AP, *et al.* Assessment of elderly people in general practice. 1: social circumstances and mental state. *British Journal of General Practice* 1991; **41**: 9–12.

4 Iliffe S, Gallivan S, Haines AP, *et al.* Assessment of elderly people in general practice. 2: functional abilities and medical problems. *British Journal of General Practice* 1991; **41**;13–15.

5 Brown K, Williams E, & Groom L Health checks on patients 75 years and over in Nottinghamshire after the new GP contract. *British Medical Journal* 1992; **305**: 619–21.

6 Chew CA, Wilkin D, & Glendinning C Annual assessments of patients aged 75 years and over: general practitioners' and nurses' views and experience. *British Journal of General Practice* 1994; **44**: 263–7.

7 Vetter NJ, Lewis PA, & Llewellyn G. Is there a right age for case-finding in elderly people? *Age & Ageing* 1993; **22**: 121–4.

8 Hunt SM, McKenna J, McEwen J, *et al.* The Nottingham Health Profile: subjective health status and medical consultations. *Social Science & Medicine* 1981; **15A**: 221–9.

9 Taylor R & Ford G Inequalities in old age: an examination of age, sex and class differences in a sample of community elderly. *Ageing & Society* 1983; **3**: 2.

10 Falconer J, Naughton BJ, Hughes SL, *et al.* Self-reported functional status predicts change in level of care in independent living residents of a continuing care community. *Journal of the American Geriatricians Society* 1992; **40**: 255–8.

11 Barber JH, Wallis JB, & McKeating E A postal screening questionnaire in preventive geriatric care. *Journal of the Royal College of General Practitioners* 1980; **30**: 49–51.

12 Taylor R, Ford G, & Barber H *The elderly at risk.* Research Perspectives on Ageing No.6, Age Concern Research Unit 1983.

13 Freer CB Consultation-based screening of the elderly in general practice: a pilot study. *Journal of the Royal College of General Practitioners* 1987; **37**: 455–6.

14 Iliffe S, See Tai S, Haines A, *et al.* Are the elderly alone an at-risk group? *British Medical Journal* 1992; **305**: 1001–4.

15 Iliffe S, Haines A, Stein A, *et al.* Assessment of elderly people in general practice. 3: confiding relationships and depression. *British Journal of General Practice* 1992; **41**: 459–61.

16 Lindley CM, Tully MP, Paramsothy V, *et al.* Inappropriate medication is a major cause of adverse drug reactions in elderly patients. *Age & Ageing* 1992; **21**: 294–300.

17 Gerson L W, Jarjoura D, & McCord G Risk of imbalance in elderly people with impaired hearing or vision. *Age & Ageing* 1989; **18**: 31–4.

18 Baker S P Harvey AH Fall injuries in the elderly. Clin.Geriatr.Med. 1985; **1**: 501–12

19 MacCuish AC Who should screen for diabetic retinopathy? *Diabetes Reviews* 1992; **1**(1): 5–8.

20 Stephens SDG, Callaghan DE , Hogan S, *et al.* Hearing disability in people aged 50–65. *British Medical Journal* 1990; **300**: 508–11.

21 Hickish G Hearing problems of elderly people. *British Medical Journal* 1989; **299**: 1415–6.

22 Grimby A, Milson I, Mollander U, *et al.* The influence of urinary incontinence on the quality of life of elderly women. *Age & Ageing* 1992; **22**: 82–9.

23 Ekelund P & Rundgren A Urinary incontinence in the elderly with implications for hospital care consumption and social disability. *Arch. Gerontol. Geriatr.* 1987; **6**: 11–18.

24 Snape J Castleden C M, Duffin H, *et al.* Long-term follow-up of habit retraining for bladder instability in elderly patients. *Age & Ageing* 1989; **18**: 192–4.

25 Jolleys J Reported prevalence of urinary incontinence in women in a general practice. *British Medical Journal* 1988; **296**: 1300–2.

26 Strawbridge W J, Kaplan G A, Camacho T *et al.* The dynamics of disability and functional change in an elderly cohort. *Journal of the American Geriatricians Society* 1992; **40**: 799–806.

27 Iliffe S, Gould MM, Mitchley S, *et al.* Evaluation of brief screening instruments for dementia, depression and problem drinking in general practice. *British Journal of General Practice*, 1994; **44**: 503–7.

28 Walters K, Iliffe S, Orrell M, *et al.* Discovering unmet need in older people: a pilot study of a new needs assessment tool . WONCA/EGPRW Conference, Majorca, May 22–24th 1999.

29 Sidell M *Health in old age: myth, mystery and management* . Open University Press, Buckingham 1995.

30 Wenger GC *Old people's health and experience of caring services.* Liverpool University Press, Liverpool 1988.

31 Haug M & Lavin B *Consumerism in medicine: challenging physician authority* . Sage, London 1983.

32 Thorne SE & Robinson CA Guarded alliance: health care relationships in chronic illness. *Imag. J. Nurs. Sch.* 1989; **21**(3): 153–7.

33 Coppard LC *Self health care and older people: a manual for public policy and programme development.* WHO, Copenhagen 1984.

34 Stuck AE, Siu AL, Wieland GD, *et al.* Effects of a comprehensive geriatric assessment on survival, residence and function: a meta-analysis of controlled trials. *Lancet* 1993; **342**: 1032–6.

35 Rich MW, Beekham V, Wittenberg C, *et al.* A multidisciplinary intervention to prevent the readmission of elderly patients with congestive heart failure. *New England Journal of Medicine* 1995; **333**: 1190–5.

36 Stuck AE, Aronow HU, Steiner A, *et al.* A trial of annual in-home comprehensive geriatric assessment for elderly people living in the community. *New England Journal of Medicine* 1995; **333**: 1184–9.

37 Tinetti ME, Inouye SK, Gill TM, *et al.* Shared risk factors for falls, incontinence and functional dependence. *Journal of the American Medical Association* 1995; **273**: 1348–53.

38 Beck JC & Stuck A preventing disability: beyond the black box. *Journal of the American Medical Association* 1996; **276**: 1756–7.

39 Walker A *The care gap.* Local Government Information Unit, London 1985.

40 Gray A M, Whelan A, & Normand C *Care in the community: a study of services and costs in six districts.* Centre for Health Economics, University of York 1988.

41 Walker A Community care: past, present and future. In Iliffe S & Munro J (eds) *Healthy choices: future options for the NHS*, Lawrence & Wishart, London 1997.

42 Walker A Community care. In McCarthy M (ed) *The new politics of welfare.* Macmillan London, 1989.

43 Walker A (ed) *Community care.* Basil Blackwell, Oxford,1982.

44 Smith CW The geography of private residential care. In Morgan K (ed) *Gerontology: responding to an ageing society.* Jessica Kingsley, London 1992.

45 Day P & Klein R the business of welfare. *New Society* 1987; **19 June**: 11–13.

46 Audit Commission *Making a reality of community care.* PSI, London 1986.

47 Bradshaw J *Financing private care for the elderly.* Department of Social Policy and Social Work, University of York 1988.

48 Griffiths R *Community care: agenda for action.* A report to the Secretary for State for Social Services, HMSO, London 1988.

49 Davies B Resources, needs and outcomes in community services – why academic caution is useful. In Morgan K (ed) *Gerontology: responding to an ageing society.* Jessica Kingsley, London 1992.

50 *Caring for people: community care in the next decade and beyond.* Cmnd 849, HMSO, London 1989.

51 Leedham I, & Wistow G *Community care and general practitioners: The role of GPs in the assessment process, with special reference to the perspectives of social services departments.* Nuffield Institute Working Papers, 1–44, 1992.

52 Hudson B Breaks in the chain. *Health Services Journal* 1994; **April 24.**

53 Lloyd M, Webb S, & Singh S Community care reforms: early implications for general practice. *British Journal of General Practice* 1994; **44:** 338–9.

54 Samuel OW & Dodge D A course in collaboration for social workers and general practitioners. *Journal of the Royal College of General Practitioners* 1981; **31:** 172–5.

55 Thomas RV & Corney RH Working with community mental health professionals: a survey among general practitioners. *British Journal of General Practice* 1993; **43:** 417–21.

56 Qureshi H & Walker A *The caring relationship.* Macmillan, London 1989.

57 Walker A, Guillemard A-M, & Alber J *Older people in europe – social and economic policies.* European Commission, Brussels 1993.

58 Walker A *Age and attitudes.* European Commission, Brussels 1993.

59 Davies B, Bebbington A, & Charnley H *Resources, needs and outcomes in community-based care.* Avebury, Aldershot 1990.

60 Bowl R Social work with old people. In Phillipson C &. Walker A (eds) *Ageing and social policy.* Aldershot, Gower 1986.

61 Walker C Older people or people with developmental disabilities, *Ageing and Society* 1998; **19**(4): 505–16.

CHAPTER THREE

A new direction?

A systematic approach to the functional and health assessment of older people in the community is needed, but as we have shown the 1990 contractual obligation as presently configured does not appear to meet this need. The appraisal carried out in 1996 for the NHS Executive[1] showed how little progress had been made in developing a preventive and proactive approach to primary care for older people after the phase of innovation was interrupted by the imposition of the new contract. The findings of this appraisal make disappointing reading, but they do indicate some ways forward for primary health care . Similar attempts to overcome the problems of reorganized social care, in favour of joint working, have produced interesting innovations that might become models for the future.

The 75-and-over checks

The 1996 appraisal did identify some examples of 'good practice' from which all primary care teams can learn, but there was no single model that appeared to be easily reproducible. The three main models of good practice which emerged were, in order in decreasing frequency:

(1) **GP led, with nurse support.** The general practitioners designed the assessment programme but delegated its implementation to practice or community nurses, or to health care assistants. These programmes tended to follow the themes of the contractual obligation (see Chapter 2), but with little standardization in their approach and limited use of valid assessment tools. The assessments done in one practice, or by one individual, would not necessarily be the same as those done elsewhere, or by different professionals, creating uncertainty about the meaning of the information gleaned from any patient.
(2) **Nurse or profession allied to medicine (PAM) led, with GP support.** The general practitioners provided medical input to an assessment process that had been developed by nurses or health visitors. These assessments

46

tended to be better grounded in standardized methods, and used tools like the Barthel index for measuring functional ability which had been brought in from the nursing or physiotherapy repertoire.

(3) **Multidisciplinary team assessments** using a 'one-stop shop' approach involving different professional groups in a patient-centred process, so that older patients saw (say) a nurse, a physiotherapist, and a chiropodist in a single visit that sometimes had as much a social function as a clinical one. Funding for these expensive services seemed precarious, although they appeared popular with patients and staff, and at first glance efficient in their concentration of resources.

Innovation was uncommon, as was a consistent approach, compared with a simple delegation of check-list assessment. However, despite the disappointing impact of the 75-and-over checks five years after their introduction, there were common features from each of these models which appear to be particularly effective in routine use, including:

- approaches that were made initially by letter, enclosing a questionnaire to be completed by the patient or, where necessary, their carer
- use of agreed criteria for the identification of 'caseness' and the follow-up of questionnaire responses
- a mechanism to follow up non-responders, by telephone, flagging records for later opportunistic reminders, or even home visiting
- use of clear referral guidelines for common problems like visual loss or depression.

A social approach to health assessment of older people had survived the reduction of tasks to a check-list. In these different models the perceived benefits of the screening programme included both identifying unmet need, particularly on the initial assessment, and simply making a link with the 75+ age group, informing its members about the kinds of services available, should they be required.

More problematic issues raised by staff involved in these different approaches included the following:

(1) **Ownership.** Although most checks were carried out by nurses, they were not usually instrumental in setting up the service. This is not surprising since the contractual obligation is with the GP, but it can create problems if the nurse disagrees with the format and content of the assessment. Similarly, if the service is dependent on one significant person for its survival, it may lose impetus when that person is not there, and the morale of staff engaged in carrying out the checks can fall when the 'prime mover' is no longer in post. Where a team approach is used to set up and carry out the checks, this problem is avoided.

(2) **Where to assess – home or surgery**. Opinions were divided among those involved in this work as to where the patient is most appropriately assessed. Many of the staff involved thought that it was important to see the patient in their own environment in order to gain the maximum

amount of information, but the checks carried out in patients' homes usually took considerably longer, partly because of travelling time. Other staff emphasized the need to be efficient with staff time and argued strongly for the patient coming to the surgery or health centre where they could be seen by all the necessary personnel on one site.

(3) **When to assess.** There was considerable interest amongst those already undertaking 75-and-over checks in the idea of starting some kind of screening for those aged 65 and over, but resource limitations prevented most staff from implementing this. There was evidence, however, that where premises and resources were available, health and social services professionals were trying to set up services aimed at this younger age group.

(4) **How to assess**. The focus of the check varied between practices. In some the emphasis for the routine check was on a social and functional assessment; in others the check had more of a medical focus. The type and use of screening instruments also varied enormously.

(5) **Local residential and nursing homes**. There were mixed feelings about the appropriateness of staff from the practice or community nursing services carrying out the 75-and-over checks in nursing homes in particular. Many felt that they were interfering when the patient's needs were already being met by qualified staff and there was also some feeling that it was a waste of their time. However, in some areas there was the concern that these were exactly the elderly people who may 'slip through the net', especially where there were high proportions of untrained staff or an impermanent workforce in residential and nursing homes who did not know the residents very well.

(6) **Who does the assessment?** Although most of the screening was carried out by nurses, their training and experience was highly variable. Those with greater experience or with 'nurse practitioner' training often took on a more medical role, for example by initiating investigations. Others, either with less experience or with some reluctance to move into this arena, referred such cases to the GP. There was some evidence that, in order to avoid missing some pathology, routine blood tests and other minor investigations were carried out on all those seen. The benefits to the patients of such a defensive approach were not clear.

One respondent in this appraisal, a district nurse in a fundholding practice with a nursing team in which district nurses, health visitors, and practice nurses assessed the over-75s, commented:

'At present there appears to be neither a uniform cohesive approach to providing these checks nor an agreed aim. The different nursing groups appear to have different objectives and understandings of what should be included at assessment. Our local health promotion agency has not responded, to date [April 1996], with advice regarding content for assessment'.

The models of service organization developed to deliver these assessments, and the concerns of staff around the implementation of an assessment programme, seemed much the same five years after the introduction of the 75-and-over checks as they were five years or more before. The absence of progress, and the lack of new ideas for working with older patients, are striking. This is not for lack of models and methods, as we shall demonstrate in Chapters 11 and 12, but for lack of resources, leadership within general practice, and commitment within the NHS administration. Far from rolling out a tried and tested programme of useful and effective health promotion for older people, the 75-and-over checks appear to have blocked innovation and experimentation to find the best approaches to anticipatory care in later life.

The 'top-down' approach exemplified by the 1990 contract has failed to improve the quality of primary care for older people, and the problems identified in the 1995/6 appraisal reinforce the need for an alternative approach. One such approach could be to reduce the assessment screening programme to the minimum intervention supported by existing evidence of effectiveness. Another would be to adopt a conscious, systematized case-finding and case management approach, making maximum use of the information technology available to primary care teams, whilst explicitly addressing the issues of ownership, teamworking and the process described above.

A minimal screening programme

Two medical actions can make an immediate difference to the health of older people: annual influenza vaccination (supported by immunization against pneumococcal pneumonia) and control of hypertension. Both of these should be programmes that practices should implement as part of a package of health promotion activity, and review critically in their annual reports. Annual influenza vaccination is cheap, largely acceptable, and reduces the incidence of and mortality from, major respiratory tract infections in older people.[2]

Treatment of hypertension at all ages up to 80 reduces the incidence of and mortality from, both heart disease and stroke, although GPs will need consciously to overcome a bias towards treating younger rather than older patients if these benefits are to be obtained.[3] The benefits of hypertension management in the age group 65–80 are discussed in detail in Chapter 7. Existing electronic medical records allow the uptake of influenza immunization and the extent and effectiveness of hypertension case-finding and treatment in older people to be managed and audited relatively easily.

Five other common problems for older people could usefully be considered by primary care teams as themes for their work, but only in the context of evaluation of different approaches:[4]

(1) Osteoporosis, where dietary and vitamin D supplementation appear to be effective, and screening using DEXA scanning appears to be sufficiently sensitive and specific to warrant further evaluation. We will return to the topic of osteoporosis in Chapter 5.
(2) Iatrogenesis, where medication review and patient education can reduce the number of avoidable admissions to hospital with problems caused or

exacerbated by inappropriate prescribing, drug interactions, or excessive drug dosages. This is a matter of great importance where action at practice level can have immediate beneficial effects, and we will discuss it further in this chapter.

(3) Depression, where case-finding, counselling, and social engagement offer some prospects for reducing the burden of morbidity. A fuller review of this subject appears in Chapter 9.

(4) Urinary incontinence, where case-finding and case management may be effective in improving quality of life. The topic of incontinence is dealt with in Chapter 8.

(5) Accidents, where home modifications appear effective in reducing the frequency and seriousness of accidents. This issue is discussed in more detail in Chapter 5.

Iatrogenesis is a major clinical issue in the community, particularly for older people. The growth in the effectiveness and range of medication available for an ageing population has made medical treatment for the disorders of later life into a problem for GPs. The GP contract is not specific about the exact nature of the 'medication review' required in the 75-and-over check, and because of the impact of early studies GP attention has tended to focus on repeat prescribing with its attendant loss of regime flexibility and its potential for prescribing errors, drug interaction, and inadvertent overdosage.[5,6] Inappropriate prescribing of the wrong medication for the wrong condition is also implicated in iatrogenesis, whilst issues around undertreatment of older people with established disease have been less prominent in debates about the medical care of older people.

Box 3.1 *Key messages about a minimalist programme*

Existing evidence about prevention of ill health and disability supports the following actions:

- influenza and pneumococcus vaccination
- hypertension case-finding and treatment.

Other clinical problems where systematic assessment may be justified include:

- osteoporosis screening, and treatment
- medication review, focused on polypharmacy
- depression, to identify individuals with major depression
- urinary incontinence
- home accidents causing injury.

In addition, contextual information on social, enviromental, and economic circumstances are important in offering advice, information, or referral to other services and community provision in response to the identification of clinical problems. Offering signposts and guidance through the variety of health, local authority, and voluntary sector services is an important function linked to case management, as we discuss below.

Repeat prescribing

Drug adverse effects and iatrogenic disorders are particularly common amongst older people needing urgent admission to in-patient care. Between 6% and 10% of older people admitted to acute hospital beds have iatrogenic disorders, variously attributed to multiple prescribing for multiple pathology, problems of compliance, changes in pharmacokinetics and pharmacodynamics, and inappropriate prescribing.[7] Changes in pharmacokinetics and pharmacodynamics can be significant for some older patients, but often can be avoided by dose reductions.[8] The number of prescribed drugs received is associated with increasing age and increasing numbers of diseases and disabilities,[9] but whilst multiple prescribing increases the risk of drug interactions, these cause only a small proportion of adverse drug reactions.[7]

Age as such does not appear to affect compliance with treatment regimes, which is related to:

- knowledge about the medication
- belief in the importance of taking medication
- understanding what the prescribing doctor has said
- less fear of illness
- being able to read the label on the medication container.[10]

Treatment regimes may be changed by older patients because of lack of information about new drugs, especially after hospital discharge,[11] and the authority and influence of the original prescriber as well as dependence on some medicines may prolong drug use inappropriately.[12] However, the commonest cause of adverse drug reactions in older people appears to be prescription of the wrong medication,[7] causing perhaps half of all acute admissions for iatrogenesis.[8]

Inappropriate prescribing

Most inappropriate prescribing arises in general practice, where the volume of patient contact is greatest. GPs may have limited or dated education in therapeutics, and the main supplier of postgraduate education in therapeutics may still be the pharmaceutical industry, even though prescribing rationality is a physician characteristic negatively associated with reliance on information from drug firms.[13] Relative isolation from other professional influences, and an inability to focus in depth on one area of therapeutics because of the generalist nature of practice, may make prescribing a problematic area to control and change. Feedback about prescribing may make at least short-term differences to medication use by older patients, especially when provided by pharmacists,[14] but pessimists will argue that audits of prescribing only change prescribing habits amongst the auditors.[15]

However, a balanced view of drug prescribing in general practice and of medication use by older people puts the problem of iatrogenesis into perspective. Freer demonstrated that 42% of older patients in general practice received no regular medication, and that only 17% had three or more medi-cines prescribed regularly.[16] Cartwright found that while over a third of older people were taking prescribed drugs of which their GPs were unaware, over 80% of the drugs reported were being taken appropriately.[17] The problem of iatrogenic disorders is seen most clearly from the hospital vantage point, where the relatively small numbers of people affected are concentrated, acces-sible for investigation, and amenable to control and supervision of their med-ication use. This is not an argument for dismissing the issue as unimportant– on the contrary, its small scale for GPs makes it easier to manage and modify.

British GPs are in a better position to reduce inappropriate prescribing than doctors in many other countries because of their role as gatekeeper to special-ist services. North American experience, for example, shows that the risk of potentially inappropriate drug combinations increases with the number of physicians involved in the medical management of older people.[18] Working in teams may also increase prescribing rationality, with less inappropriate pre-scribing occurring when multidisciplinary primary care teams provide care for older people,[19] although this has not yet been demonstrated in UK settings.

Early research into prescribing for older patients within general practice, reviewed by Knox, identified a number of issues, including:

- the need to distinguish between 'realistic' and 'rational' prescribing
- uncertainty about the extent and significance of adverse effects
- the need to reduce prescribing of particular groups of medicines – for example, hypnotics.[20]

The difference between rational and realistic prescribing is probably the most important of these issues, in terms of understanding prescribing in gen-eral practice. Rational prescribing can occur when the prescriber:

- knows exactly what medical problem is being treated
- understands how a chosen medication works and how it will alter the identified problem,
- understands what potential interactions are possible, either with other drugs or with other, co-existent illnesses.

Hospital specialists are in a good position to prescribe rationally because they usually know what condition they are treating, tend to have in-depth knowledge of a narrow range of disorders and their treatments, and have access to sources of information about medication such as other team mem-bers and hospital pharmacists. Prescribing in general practice differs from that in hospital medicine because there is often greater uncertainty about diag-noses in the community, when people often present with problems and symp-toms that are not easily categorized. In older people multiple symptoms that are not easy to attribute may co-exist with several known medical problems, some with a range of potential consequences or expressions. Prescribing may be 'realistic' in the sense that it is aimed at symptom-relief in the absence of a diagnosis, or even at hypothesis testing to reach a diagnosis, without being 'rational' in the clinical–pharmacological sense.[21]

For example, older patients complaining of dizziness may have neurological, cardiovascular or psychological causes for their symptom, but distinguishing between them by clinical examination may be difficult in the primary care setting, so that GPs may opt to treat the most likely cause to relieve symptoms and confirm the diagnosis. Similarly, pain in the lower back, or in hip and knee joints, may be treated with non-steroidal anti-inflammatory analgesics (NSAIDs) even though its origin may not be in inflammatory joint disease, but in sciatic nerve compression, osteoarthritis, or even depression.

In general practice, brief contacts with large numbers of people whose medical problems are less clearly delineated may make iatrogenic disorder a more difficult problem to address, especially if most realistic prescribing does no harm or even appears to do good. A clearer picture of the nature of GP prescribing for older patients which puts these problems into perspective requires studies of whole populations.

Community studies

Two community studies have demonstrated the extent of medication use by older people, and offer a different perspective on problems of prescribing usually identified from the hospital vantage point. Cartwright and Smith interviewed a representative sample of 805 people aged 65 and over drawn from electoral registers in 10 parliamentary constituencies, in the early 1980s, reviewing both the drugs prescribed and their usage.[21]

The Two Boroughs study interviewed at home and reviewed the medication of a random sample of those aged 75 and over, recruited from the age–sex registers of nine practices in working-class districts of north London in 1987–1988.[22] All people aged 75 and over registered with the practices were asked to participate in a study of health problems in older people, and a 90% response rate was obtained. A random one in five sample (n=231) were interviewed in depth in their homes, and medication being used by 221 of them was checked by the interviewer.

Only two-thirds of those studied (n=148, 67%) were taking prescribed medication, less than the 75% reported by Williamson in 1978[23] and the 80% reported by Knox in 1980.[20] One or two prescribed medicines were being taken by 83 people (38%) and 65 (29%) were taking three or more. The factors associated with no use of prescribed medication in the Two boroughs study were:

- male sex
- normal cognitive function (mini-Mental State Examination scores of 25– 30)
- few diagnoses in the GP medical record
- little or no contact with medical or other services in the previous three months
- high levels of reported functional activity.

The patterns of medication use found in these two community studies are shown in table 3.1.

Where medication was being taken the patterns of use were similar in the two studies. The differences in use of beta-blockers and hypnotics may represent changes in prescribing habits or may be survivor effects in different cohorts. Prescribing of cardiovascular system drugs increased, with increased prescribing of angiotensin-converting enzyme (ACE) inhibitors and calcium channel-blockers; hypnotic and tranquillizer use fell, reflecting the efforts made to change prescribing habits in general practice.

Undertreatment

The very real concerns about iatrogenesis, and the problems of repeat prescribing that may promote polypharmacy and inappropriate medication use, have overshadowed another important problem, the undertreatment of disease in older patients by general practitioners. Undertreatment of common conditions like hypertension, heart disease, chronic obstructive pulmonary disease (COPD), diabetes, and depression appears to be a major contributor to the morbidity and mortality associated with these disorders. Two recent studies of aspirin and anticoagulant use in older patients with cardiovascular disease which have demonstrated the extent of this problem, and its implications for the health of the ageing population, are discussed in Chapter 7. Similarly, failure to treat remediable disorders can provoke inappropriate institutionalization or increase dependency of those already living in nursing or residential homes.[24]

One of the important tasks facing PCGs is to deal with undertreatment of older

Table 3.1 *Community studies of medicine use by older people*

Proportions of older people using prescribed medication on a regular basis, by drug group

	Cartwright & Smith (65 & over) n=805	Two Boroughs study ** (75 & over) n=221
Diuretics	25%	22%
NSAIDs	15%	13%
Hypnotics & tranquillizers	15%	8%
Beta-blockers	11%	5%
Digoxin	6%	8%

* *Cartwright A & Smith C Elderley people: their medicines and their doctors. Routledge, London 1988.*
** *Iliffe S, Gallivan S, Haines A P et al. Assessment of elderly people in general practice: medication use amongst community-dwelling older people. (Unpublished data.)*

people, remembering that a review of medication alone may not necessarily help with the untreated patient with atrial fibrillation, nor even the older person with heart disease not receiving aspirin. A broader approach to case management of older patients is needed, in which the evidence about optimal care is brought to bear on each patient. Collating the evidence on a wide range of conditions and putting it into practice in a systematic way for whole populations is a sizeable problem, but one way to begin it is through case management of individuals receiving multiple medicines. We will return to the topic of case management soon, but note now how reviewing medication is a route into a more complex process.

The role for community geriatricians in collating and updating the evidence needed to prescribe rationally for older people may be large, and their involvement in case management as expert advisors may allow fruitful collaboration between primary care staff and hospital specialists to increase, particularly at a time when the organization of primary care is changing rapidly. Team care appears to reduce the risk of inappropriate prescribing[20] and may be shown to reduce undertreatment too, so the next step in the development of primary care for older people may be to extend existing teamwork to include the necessary specialist expertise for systematic care of older people.

Medication review

The research of Cartwright and Smith generated recommendations to improve prescribing for older people, including:

- regular audit by all general practices
- improve documentation of prescribing, particularly at hospital discharge, and of risk factors, over-the-counter medicine use, and adverse effects
- routine inspection of drug supplies at every consultation.[25]

Tallis proposed simple rules for prescribing: develop a limited range of drug therapies that are well understood; consult reliable information sources; consider non-drug management of problems; make risk–benefit considerations explicit to the patient; adjust doses rationally, remembering the unpredictability of pharmacokinetics and pharmacodynamics in older people; and monitor long-term medication use for both efficacy and adverse effects.[8]

Computerization of general practice medical records makes these recommendations feasible, although existing software may not identify all significant interactions.[26] However, the best approach to medication review remains unclear, and more detailed guidance is necessary so that GPs can focus their attention on those individuals most likely to suffer serious adverse effects or iatrogenic problems from prescribed medication. If the problem is perceived to be mainly one of polypharmacy and its consequences then the approach is easy, and begins with a computer search of repeat medication. If the issue is seen differently, as one of inappropriate prescribing, it is harder to tackle because every prescription is a potential candidate for review. Here the community studies can help practitioners to prioritize patients and problems for review, and demonstrate the value of this kind of primary care research.

The section of the Two Boroughs study which yielded information on medicine use involved 239 people aged 75 and over, which is equivalent to the elderly population of an average two-doctor practice of about 4000 people. Only 65 individuals were taking three or more prescribed medicines and could be considered as experiencing polypharmacy, and being at greatest risk from inadvertent drug interactions. Reviewing this number of high-risk patients would entail only one medication review per doctor per week, which is a small and realistic objective. Repeat prescribing managed by computer allows scope for automatic detection of at least some potential drug interactions and morbidity contraindications to prescribing, so that the doctor is able to focus on the risks and benefits of treatment. Other issues can then also be addressed, including the impact of age and cognitive function on understanding of drug use,[27] and simple, important but often neglected details lsuch as drug labelling and patients' ability to open drug containers and packs.[28] It has been apparent for over 20 years that community pharmacists can contribute a great deal of expertise to this review process.[13, 29]

Prescribing patterns can be changed if particularly problematic groups of drugs are targeted and alternative forms of treatment sought. Non-steroidal drugs are one example, where the benefits of treatment may be slight and the potential hazards great. Digoxin or diuretics may be other drugs that could usefully become the focus of attention at practice level because of the tendency for their overuse,[30] their potential for interaction, the tendency to under-monitor their effects,[31] and their metabolic cost.[32]

Finally, diagnoses may need review before medicines, but here the problems of rational and realistic prescribing remain complex. For example, treatment of symptoms of depression may seem inappropriate, but effective treatment of later-life depression is limited to the severe forms of the condition, where untreated mortality is high.[33] Most older people with depression have less severe forms and the effectiveness of different therapies and treatments for these lower severity levels of depression is unknown.[34] General practitioners may have to choose between prescribing antidepressants that themselves produce adverse effects or even iatrogenic disorders to depressed older people, or opting for symptom-relief that seems more acceptable to the ill individual. The solution to these problems may lie with better identification of those depressed elderly people who would most benefit from antidepressant treatment (perhaps using validated screening scales), and with research into alternative, non-pharmaceutical forms of treatment for those with less severe depression. These issues will be reviewed in Chapter 9.

Given the limitations of our knowledge about illness in the community, the lack of effective responses to common problems, and the time constraints within which GPs must work, some inappropriate prescribing (when viewed with hindsight) may persist. However, the extent of inappropriate prescribing can be reduced by focusing medication review on the key drug groups that generate iatrogenesis, and by seeking non-drug solutions to some problems.

The case-finding approach we have described for identifying those at risk of iatrogenic disorders applies to diagnosing hypertension, cataract detection, and other common, treatable problems of later life surveyed in this book. Such a minimalist approach does not require screening of the whole population, and is amenable to opportunistic approaches. However, once found, 'cases' need management, particularly when they have multiple medical, psychological, and social problems. Such case mangement is a major task, requiring time, effort, and skill, and we will discuss it in some detail here before returning to it in Chapter 11.

Case management

As we argued in Chapter 2, case management looks important to the development of optimal primary medical care for older people, but its origins in the USA make its exact significance for British circumstances unclear. We have a view on the nature of case management, but it is a term that has been used in different ways by different disciplines, and we will first explore these differences to reveal some of the cultural differences between the professional groupings engaged in primary care. Most health professionals would conceptualize a process of case or care management in terms of their own activities. This process includes gathering information, identifying problems, applying their professional knowledge and personal experience to these problems, planning a course of action, acting on that plan, and then reviewing their efforts. Doctors are more likely to describe their activities as 'case' management and the nurses as 'care' management, highlighting their different perspectives of their task.

In health and social care systems, the term 'case management' is a relatively recent concept , emerging in the late 1970s in North America. There it was primarily a response to the increasing fragmentation of services and their spiralling costs.[35] Components of case management included assessment, diagnosis, service planning , implementation, and most importantly coordination and monitoring service delivery. Throughout the eighties and nineties case management came to be seen as an integral part of the American system of 'managed care', by which the health care of individual patients is financed according to detailed clinical protocols and therapy specifications. Case management in this context has a role as a cost-containment mechanism, akin the the British GP's gatekeeper role. The diversity of American models of case management reflects the diversity of funding systems and of clinical services, including direct care providers, case management companies, and insurance companies.[36] Most of these models focus on service utilization by individual patients but some provide more comprehensive approaches to populations.[37]

At first glance it is difficult to see how this American substitute for the gatekeeper role of general practice could apply to the British setting, but it did offer a model for services without such a role, in social care. The application of case management methods in social services in the UK during the eighties, particularly through the work of the Personal Social Services Research Unit at the University of Kent,[38] led to its advocacy in the Griffiths Report and adoption in the NHS and Community Care Act 1990 (see Chapter 2). The focus of this approach was very clearly on promoting mechanisms of coordination between health services, social services, and housing organizations, and the term 'care management' was adopted because it was the care, not the person (i.e. the case), that was being managed.

Subsequently the term 'care management' has been used in the UK almost exclusively in the context of the organizational system associated with the provision of the very community care that has proved so problematic. The term 'care manager' is applied to the local authority employee with responsibility for assessing, planning, and ensuring the provision of care. The legislation and accompanying national guidance placed care management both at the level of the individual's care and at a macro level of a system to manage the care of groups of individuals.

This may be confusing to practitioners, and it may therefore be helpful to view case and care management as part of a spectrum of activity built on a cyclical process of review, action, review, with case management (of people) being medical and care management (of services) being more typical of social services and, sometimes, of nursing care. We are arguing that a more proactive model of anticipatory care would use a case management model. By this we mean reviewing the health status and health care provided for an individual, seeking to apply evidence-based guidelines to promote best practice, and checking that simple but important issues such as checking blood pressure, offering influenza immunization, and screening for cognitive impairment are not missed. Care management is not dismissed because as we shall show it has an important impact on the support given to older patients, but it is not the best option for health care that focuses on individuals and their needs before populations and theirs.

Such a case management approach can be systematic in four ways:

(1) by reviewing all aspects of an individual's health against a check-list of common problems amenable to medical or nursing intervention (this differs from the current 75-and-over checks because caseness is defined more precisely by use of standardized assessment tools)

(2) by involving different disciplines to give different perspectives on each individual's problems and situation, in a similar way to the case conferences of social care or the team meetings of geriatric medicine

(3) by following up decisions taken and plans made to ensure that action is taken and that the patient benefits, using the practice's electronic medical record as the basis for a review system analagous to the 'call and recall' approach to cervical cytology screening and mammography

(4) by providing guidance, referral, advocacy, and follow-up through the health, local authority, and voluntary sector services which can best address the elements of the health problems that are outside the scope of primary health care.

When 80-year-old Mrs G. the Shakespeare buff, responded to an invitation to a 75-and-over check, the practice nurse reacted to her complaint that her left leg hurt by asking her about her sleeping pattern, because the nurse knew that per-

sistent pain and depression were linked, and that depression and sleep disturbance often occurred together. Mrs G. admitted that she slept all afternoon but
found sleeping at night difficult. The nurse took an alcohol history, using a simple quantity–frequency question, and found out that Mrs G. estimated a weekly
intake of 20 units. The nurse then obtained Mrs G.'s agreement to work through
the 15-item Geriatric Depression Scale (15GDS), which gave a score of 9, above
the usual depression threshold. She talked to Mrs G.'s doctor, who remembered
her husband's death some 10 years previously from multi-infarct dementia, and
what a difficult person he had been. He decided to invite Mrs G. for a second
check, this time concentrating on her apparent depression and the specific
symptoms of pain in the leg.

This approach is similar to the Comprehensive Geriatric Assessment
(CGA) with follow-up that appears to be capable of reducing the burden of
disability, but is applied on a case-by-case basis rather than to whole populations. Systematic case management of the CGA type has been shown to be
effective in reducing hospital admission rates and producing positive health
gain in North American settings.[39] It may be important that it can be led and
coordinated by nurses, not doctors, thus maintaining the delegation of functions begun with the 75-and-over assessments, but with the nurse in more of
a decision-making, leadership role.

To be effective, systematic case management requires reliable information
that is easy to access and a body of knowledge to support clinical decision-
making. The electronic medical record can be the basis for a comprehensive
profile of the health and functional ability of older people, so that individual-
ized strategies for intervention can be generated and recorded easily, and the
impact of case management measured. We will return to the issue of information systems in Chapter 4. Guidelines on management approaches for different conditions are needed because they have been shown to improve the
quality of clinical care when used by practice teams within a review process.[41]

With the current drive towards evidence-based medicine there is increasing
pressure on clinicians to use clinical guidelines to aid in decision-making and
help direct their management. Evidence exists that guidelines can be effective
in changing health professionals' behaviour when used in combination with
educational intervention strategies or feedback mechanisms. [40–42] It is has been
shown that valid guidelines when implemented *can* lead to changes in clinical
practice and ultimately to improvements in outcomes for patients, although
guidelines alone do not guarantee change in practice. Therefore the exact role
for guidelines in everyday clinical practice remains controversial, and many
problems lie in applying the guidelines on an individual patient level. This is
particularly evident for older people who often do not fit neatly into identified
categories of single pathologies.

The numbers of available guidelines are increasing rapidly and with the
advent of the National Institute for Clinical Effectiveness (NICE) this trend
looks set to continue. But what of the quality of these guidelines? How many
of them could or should be relied upon by working practitioners faced with
the often complex problems of older patients? Older people are frequently

excluded as subjects from clinical research[43, 44]and hence it can be difficult to find good-quality research that is directly applicable to older age groups. With an increased likelihood of co-existing complex multiple pathologies, different drug absorption, metabolism, and sensitivity profiles, and higher mortality and morbidity rates, interventions may have a vastly different impact in older people. Table 3.2, derived from work done in the Case Management of Older People (COPE) trial, shows the range of age-specific guidelines applicable to older people, together with their sources, in early 1998.[45] There are not many guidelines based on robust evidence, and they do not cover the wide spectrum of disease and disability associated with advancing age.

Only 16 out of 81 guidelines identified on a wide search were soundly based on evidence with explicit methodology and contained some form of advice specific to the elderly. The problem of exclusion of older people from clinical trials is well described.[43] Guideline developers would therefore have difficulty in finding good-quality, directly applicable evidence to make recommendations based on age. This might explain at least in part the large number of guidelines that fail to make even mention of age in their advice. Hence older people again find themselves selectively excluded, which in turn could have a potentially detrimental effect on their care.

Medical practitioners are facing increasing pressure to use guidelines to aid in their decision-making, but there are difficulties in implementing this for

Table 3.2 *Guidelines identified and defined as evidence based on RCTs, meta-analyses, or systematic review with explicit methodology and containing advice specific to the elderly*

Agency for health care policy research (AHCPR)	Incontinence (1992) Acute Low Back Pain (1997)
Cochrane Library	Vitamin D & Osteoporosis (1995) Hypertension (1997)
Effective Health Care Bulletin	Benign Prostatic Hypertrophy (1995) Laxatives in the Elderly (1997) Accident Prevention (1996) Influenza (1994)
North of England Evidence-based Guidelines Group	Dementia (1998) Angina (1995)
Scottish Intercollegiate Guidelines Network (SIGN)	Colorectal Cancer (1997)
Canadian Medical Association	Hypertension (1995)
Other	Systematic Review of Elder Abuse(1997) Anticoagulation in Atrial Fibrillation (1995)

older people. Until there exists an easily accessible, comprehensive source of high-quality, evidence-based guidelines we would be cautious about the overemphasis of the role of guidelines with this age group. Primary care research groups now emerging may want to consider not only the exclusion of older people from research studies, but also the treatment of co-morbidity (a common problem in later life) as an exclusion criterion from trials, and the paucity of data on the appropriateness of stopping medication after years of use, sometimes as part of a package of prescribing multiple preparations.[46]

Box 3.2 *Key messages about clinical guidelines*

- There is currently a strong emphasis on using evidence-based guidelines in practice.
- Identifying and reviewing relevant guidelines is an extremely time con-suming process.
- Only 16 of the 81 guidelines identified in the COPE review were explicitly evidence based and contained age-related advice.
- Greater consideration should be given to older age groups both in research and guideline development.

What should clinicians do when the evidence runs out? The accumulated experience of clinicians remains a powerful, if sometimes flawed, guide to prac-tice, and with an ageing population it often complements the perspectives of social services on the importance of social support, and on the value of remedial action against disabilities and prosthetic interventions to maintain indepen-dence. The disabilities that impair everyday life for some older people may not fit neatly and exclusively into organic or social categories, and may not be the obvious responsibility of only one discipline. The endless debates in the eighties about whether bathing was a nursing or social care task are an example of this, and in some places led to absurd policies that deemed washing above the waist to be a social services function and cleanliness below the waist a task for the health service. Therefore the medical or nursing case manager must have some sense of what a care manager counterpart in social services is doing in situations where the patient's problems are complex and interrelated. The role of social services in the care of older people has changed enormously over the last decade, as we have tried to show in Chapter 2, and as PCGs develop and social policy shifts again under a new government, further changes are inevitable. 'Tearing down the Berlin Wall' between health and social care is now a policy objective, so we will review some of the attempts to do this in the early 1990s.

New developments in social care

Since 1993 different models of joint working between primary and social care have emerged, although as yet little information about them has been published in peer-reviewed journals. However, some examples of current joint-working schemes illustrate the potential for collaboration, and for the development of carefully evaluated joint working. Unlike the earlier attachment schemes, those currently running are aimed at facilitating community care for people with a physical illness or disability. We describe here four examples from Dickie's 1996 review of relationships between GPs and social services.[47]

Practice-based social work in Hereford and Worcester

An evaluation of practice-based social workers in two practices, one fundholding at the time of research and one about to become so, matched them with two control practices in similar areas which did not have attached social workers. In the two study practices, one social worker worked independently, reviewing all referrals from the practice team and deciding which to deal with himself and which to allocate to the social services department. In the other, the social worker took all referrals to his manager in the department for allocation.

The social worker who decided his own caseload attracted a referral rate that was 63% higher than the rate of referral from the control practices to their local social services department. It was also 31% higher than the referral rate to the attached social worker who took all his cases to a manager for allocation. Thus where the social worker was able to determine his own caseload, he attracted more referrals. In Table 3.3, the referrals from the practices to social services over the six-month study period in 1993–94 are compared in detail, showing how the bias against older people found earlier with GP attachment of social workers (see Chapter 2) may have been overcome with attachment of staff with a clearer and more focused job description. Although a smaller proportion of patients in the GP attachment group sought help for benefits, a much higher proportion reported benefits advice as a gain from their contact with the service, suggesting better targeting of help when the social worker is attached to the general practice. The greater proportion of high-priority cases in the attached social worker group also suggests that better case-finding is operating when the disciplines work alongside each other.

The priority ratings used by the social services department in the area were:

- **1a** – risk of serious harm or breakdown within the next five days
- **1b** – risk of serious harm or breakdown within the next three months
- **2** – serious hardship within the next three months and breakdown in the long term
- **3** – if the need is not met, the person, carer, or dependants will experience serious hardship
- **4** – if the need is not met there will be no improvement in the ordinary life of the person, carer, or dependants.

As well as increasing the referral rate to social services, the practice-based social workers also seemed to see a higher proportion of very 'needy' clients; 40% of study clients fell into priority rating 1a or b, almost twice the propor-

Table 3.3 *The Hereford and Worcester study*

	Study practices – referrals to practice -based social worker %	Control practices – referrals to social service department %
Referral rate over		
6 Months	0.67	0.51
Mean age	74	74
% female clients	63	69
Source of referral – GP	40	6
Source of referral – client		
or family	18	44
Priority rating 1a or 1b	43	23
Help requested with		
• accommodation	22	29
• finance/benefits	20	31
• home care packages	43	20
• aids/adaptions	5	10
Client owns home	49	47
Client rents home	24	40
Clients' views of help received:		
• nursing help at home	9	3
• help with housework	47	23
• help with meals	13	10
• move to a different home	29	33
• advice about benefits	53	27

tion from the control practices. Home care packages were given to 40% of study clients, again twice the proportion given to control clients.

Contracts with social services in Devon

In Ivybridge in Devon, a fundholding GP negotiated a special contract with social services,[48] during which each party learned about the mysterious working practices of the other. A facilitator from social services spent some time in the practice and the lead GP spent time meeting with social services managers. The GP noted:

'Like [hospital] consultants, social services' team leaders run teams of frequently changing staff. Rapid turnover in junior staff does not disturb continuity if the working relationship is between the general practitioner and the consultant rather than the house officer. This analogy helped us to see that our previous and unsuccessful requests for us to have a named social worker attached to the practice were unrealistic.'

The net result was a contract that stipulated turnaround working times for referrals to social services acceptable to the practice and referral protocols acceptable to the social services department. Later audits of communication showed that the information flow between the practice and the social services department had improved considerably.

Linkworkers in Wiltshire

The Wiltshire 'linkworkers' scheme is an example of a project where social services have worked very closely with the local community health care providers and health authorities. The result was coverage of over 50% of practices by care managers, known as linkworkers.[49] While all had some training from social services, they ranged in background from practices nurses to experienced social workers. This pilot was evaluated by Bath University in 1992.[50] Ten practices were involved, of differing sizes and fundholding status. Of the nine linkworkers, four were social workers, two were health visitors, one a district nurse, one was from Age Concern, and one had no professional background. Their funding source was equally varied; four linkworkers were funded by the FHSA, two by the health authority, and three by social services. The projects were widely appreciated by local GPs, one typical comment being:

'It's the first time in my professional life I can take a need, talk to [linkworker], then she comes back to me and converts that need into practical help.'

However, some social service managers did not share this enthusiasm, confirming that linkworking did increase overall social service workload. One social services care manager said:

'What [the linkworker] has really been a confirmation of is what we have always thought to be the case, that is, that many people presenting their problems to GPs at surgeries do not just have physical problems, but in many cases have entrenched social problems . . . I am not saying that this is not legitimate work for the social services department, and in many ways it could be preventative work, it is just that we are not resourced to deal with it. Consequently, [linkworker], in fostering and developing goodwill in the practice has inevitably found that she was having too much work pushed her way.'

Another commented:

The scheme has been important in developing links, but is limited and would be extremely expensive to replicate across all practices.'

A community services unit in Lyme Regis

The Lyme Community Care Unit[li] was created as a private limited company funded by two counties' health and community trusts and social services departments. The five GPs involved provided general medical care but beyond that were contracted to the Unit, which also appointed and employed all other staff.

The unit provided most community health services (e.g. accident and emergency, community mental health, physiotherapy, hospital at home) as well as social services. The social worker employed by the unit was directly accountable to the unit management, which included a non-executive board of local people actively involved in purchasing decisions. The unit purchased all the care it could not provide itself and was effectively responsible for the health and social welfare of 8000 people.

We can sum up what is currently understood about joint working in these terms:

- *physical proximity of office bases appears to promote ease of access for communication, which helps oil joint-working processes but see two points below*
- *joint working is as much about establishing professional relationships with others (e.g understanding of each other's roles, trust in each other's judgement and actions, regard for professional integrity of the other) as about robust administrative systems for flow of information*
- *there are many potential models but success depends on the same principles as laid out for teamworking – see Chapter 4 for more details.*

Process and outcomes

In most new joint working projects evaluation has focused almost exclusively on processes, not on outcomes, especially on how joint working improves communications between primary care and social services. Intuitively, effective communication seems essential to effective provision of care, if only because referrals are less likely to be lost, not made, or wrongly prioritised. This focus on communication, and the realization that social services operate a specialist services analogous to hospital medicine, creates a model with which general practitioners are familiar and puts social services on a more equal relationship with primary care. However it needs to be clearly shown that the sometimes costly methods of joint working which are being tested in different places really do improve the care for those people who use the services and represent an efficient allocation of resources.

In 1984 when Sheppard noted the lack of communication between GPs and social workers[52] he concluded:

'GPs do not consider as their responsibility the development and maintenance of contacts with other professionals. Nonetheless, they are quick to criticise others when communication is, in their view, poor.'

This conclusion is not substantiated by evidence in his paper, which suggested that when the referral came from a GP, communication was better than when it came from either a hospital team, the patient, or their family. The GP would be unlikely to even know of the other referrals, let alone initiate contact with social services about them. A more useful conclusion would have been to question whether it would be practicable to inform GPs when their patients were seen by social services. It would then have been interesting to re-audit letters and phone calls to see if this improved the flow of information back the other way, from GPs to social services. Of course this raises issues of confidentiality. One of the reasons why automatic notification to GPs of social services contact with one of their patients might not be feasible is the confidential nature of the client/social worker relationship, which may exclude the GP unless permission to communicate is granted by the patient. Nevertheless, a written notice from social services informing the GP that their patient had been referred by a discharging hospital team or a relative, with a contact name and number, might help the GP, hopefully without creating too much extra work for the social services department, as well as confirm the status and importance of social care.

A detailed, careful, and explicit negotiation process at the outset appears to be one of the important factors in developing a successful social services attachment in general practice.[53] Most problems that arise in joint-working schemes seem to be due to failure to work out exactly what each party expects of the other before the scheme begins. In some of the recent examples of joint working,[48] the process of negotiation itself, in negotiating contracts, is found to improve communication in a broad sense.

Other projects on joint working[54] have shown that brief weekly visits to a practice by a social worker improve communication. This type of initiative is less ambitious and expensive than basing a social worker in a practice, although it may also be viewed as second best by practices who would prefer 'their own' social worker.

One way of promoting joint working is to retrain members of the primary health care team to work as care managers, as in the linkworkers example from Wiltshire described above. District nurses and health visitors who work as care managers, employed by or funded through the local government, can have all the responsibilities of a social work care manager and still work with those older people who need nursing care at home.[55] Linkworkers may not narrow the gap between primary care and social services, but they do appear to provide a way of bridging it, if only by reducing duplication of effort.

Measuring the outcomes of joint working

In the Hereford and Worcester project a large number of very needy clients was uncovered in the study group, suggesting that there may be a pool of unmet need in the community that is revealed by basing a social worker in a practice. While social services obviously aim to work on a needs-led basis, this case-finding approach has cost implications. So while the practice based social work model is attractive to GPs and the primary health care team, it may be less attractive to social services as the extra cases create extra work and consume extra resources, all out of the cash-limited social services budget. As the social services manager interviewed in the linkworker evaluation said, while it may legitimate for social services to go into the community looking for need, it may not be practical.

This is an understandable perspective. However the purpose of social service departments is to consider all of the needs of their communities, and to prioritize their resources in the light of these needs. Keeping clear of sections of the community in need who do not currently utilize social services helps relieve short-term budgetary pressures, but at the price of failing to provide a needs-based service to the community as a whole. If closer working links allow sections of the community access to social services which they would otherwise not have, this is surely a good thing. The boards of PCGs contemplating merged health and social care budgets will need to decide whether funds should be transferred from health to social care, to meet the needs of an ageing population. Then outcomes of care will become more important than processes, to justify the transfer of resources.

How should we define which outcome measures to use in evaluation of innovative joint working? As well as qualitative information from interviews with service providers and users, quantitative data should be collected to assess the subsequent quality of life of patients and carers. Admission rates to residential care should be compared, as should the comparative costs of home care and residential care. Acute medical and surgical admission rates should be recorded for the two groups. By collecting this information for several different models of joint working, it should be possible to determine which models are most appropriate in which situation. If needs-led social work targeted at older people reduces NHS costs by reducing the need for acute medical or surgical care, then this must be reflected in budget allocation at PCG level.

Local design and management of initiatives provides ownership and goodwill for new services, which is important for success. However, this was also the way in which the 1970s attachment schemes started, and without meaningful evaluation they were early victims of local authorities' need to target resources.

'Much of the new approach is theory – as yet untried and untested on any large scale. Much of it is based on research projects usually run by people with high abilities and high motivations often with extra funding.' [56]

In order to ensure that the new approaches to joint working are not just another temporary phenomenon, PCG boards must ensure that current projects are adequately funded for realistic periods and are carefully evaluated.

The research questions are fundamental, for commonplace assumptions about joint working need testing if social services and primary care are to avoid the endless reorganization according to current ideas that has been so disruptive in both social care and the NHS over recent decades. In particular we need to know if collaborative working not only makes the recipient of services feel as good as the providers, but also materially alters the quality of life for older people. Should primary care nurses and doctors work from the same premises or are their patients and clients just as well off, or even better served, if the different disciplines retain separate identities and bases? Are community nurses more appropriate partners for social services than are doctors? What sorts of information needs are common to social and health care, and what are specific to each agency, or to each discipline?

A manifesto for change?

The NHS has not given priority to the development of assessment programmes for older people in the community, but this can now be remedied by:

- the development of professional training programmes relevant to both a minimal assessment package and a systematic case management approach
- encouraging practices to develop a 'base-up' approach to meeting need amongst older people, including:
- promoting experiments in joint working between social services, general practices, and specialists in medicine for older people at practice or locality level.

We have raised some of the issues around joint working in this chapter, and will return to them in Chapter 4. The 'base-up' approach is implicit in our argument about case management and we will make a community-oriented model of it explicit in Chapter 11. Professional training for assessment of older people, which the NHS has neglected for so long, needs some discussion here before we revisit it in Chapter 12. We will end this discussion with a review of important themes and an example of multidisciplinary professional education.

Professional training

Involving primary care workers in the kind of training that might change their practice is a problem according to all those who attempt it, and an especially large problem when considering a difficult and ostensibly unrewarding theme like the health of older people. Sitting in lectures by specialists is rewarded financially in UK general practice, but the evidence that it improves the health of older patients is non-existent. Adult-style learning, through a participative and problem-based approach, offers more hope for changing professional behaviour, but seems less attractive to organizers and practitioners alike.

These are conventional views, but they are mistaken. General practitioners and other primary care workers can and do participate in multidisciplinary learning, and can work on complex problems such as dementia diagnosis and management or chronic disease management with enthusiasm. How much this changes practice remains unknown, and needs to be investigated, but there are grounds for hoping that new styles of continuing education, with skill enhancement and transfer among and between disciplines, will help primary care staff to face the challenges of working with an ageing population.

One example of this is the nationwide 'Action on Alzheimer's' educational programme organized by the publisher, Excerpta Medica in 1997.[57] This involved three one-day workshops in London and one in each of 21 other cities which attracted nearly 800 participants, of whom almost 40% were GPs, and another 35% were community (district) nurses, practice nurses, or community psychiatric nurses.

A multidisciplinary editorial team developed a training programme for dementia diagnosis and management in primary care.[58] The core curriculum was drawn up by a multidisciplinary editorial group using a Delphi technique,[59] in which structured written communication between the central, collating group and members of an expert panel was used iteratively to reach a consensus about the content and structure of the curriculum. This approach has been used successfully in developing psychiatric nurse training,[60] and in establishing research priorities in clinical nursing,[61] and may be an important tool for PCGs seeking knowledge from local communities and engagement by different disciplines.

The programme was designed to maximize informed, multidisciplinary debate using adult learning methods,[62] and was divided into two parts: diagnosis including screening and early detection; and management options in dementia care. Each part was introduced by a local expert nominated by local experienced GPs, who acted as facilitators for the event. The experts' introduction was carefully scripted to cover the main themes of each topic in a standardized way in one hour, and the speakers were both briefed on the need to present a standard lecture and provided with a slide kit for their session. Key points from each presentation were reproduced in the workbook given to each participant at the beginning of the day.

After the overview presented by the local expert participants divided into multidisciplinary work groups which functioned on a focus group basis to achieve rapid independent learning, the identification of necessary knowledge and reflection on its use.[63]

Choice of work group had occurred at registration, and preferences were respected as far as possible whilst retaining a balance of professional groups within each group, since learning in an interagency environment is thought to promote multidisciplinary practice.[64, 65] The content of the programme was derived from the existing evidence base on dementia care, utilizing expertise from ongoing studies of dementia diagnosis and management in Bristol and Newcastle Universities[66] as well as published guidelines,[67] details of which appear in Chapter 9.

These workshops confirmed the correctness of an educational agenda, suggesting that attention should be paid to: i) diagnosis; ii) screening instruments; iii) referral criteria; iv) carers' problems; and v) information about support services. [68] GPs in particular had difficulties with early diagnosis, with diagnostic certainty, and with management of common problems in patients with dementia. The overall evaluation of the workshops by participants was strongly positive, despite (or perhaps because of) an intense day of small-group discussions around difficult topics.

This is only one example of an educational initiative designed to change the quality of primary care for one group of older people, and professional education is only one approach to enhancing the quality of services. In Chapter 4 we will discuss other key components of a strategy for service development, including information systems and teamworking methods.

References

1 Iliffe S, Gould MM, & Wallace P *The 75-and-over assessments in general practice: report 1*. Dept. of Primary Care & Population Sciences, Royal Free &UCL Medical School 1997.

2 Effectiveness *Bulletin Influenza vaccination and older people*. NHS Centre for Reviews and dissemination, University of York 1996; vol 2: no.1.

3 Ebrahim S & Davey Smith G *Health promotion for cardiovascular disease among older people*. Health Education Authority London 1996.

4 Ebrahim S *Tackling disease* . Paper presented at the symposium 'Towards a framework for promoting the health of older people.' Health Education Authority & Centre for Policy on Ageing, London 1996.

5 Burns B & Phillipson C *Drugs, ageing & society: social and pharmacological perspectives*. Croom Helm, Beckenham 1986.

6 Crome P ABC of poisoning: the elderly. *British Medical Journal* 1984; **289**: 546–8.

7 Lindley CM, Tully M P, Paramsothy V, *et al.* Inappropriate medication is a major cause of adverse drug reactions in elderly patients. *Age & Ageing* 1992; **21**: 294–300.

8 Tallis RC Preventing drug reactions in the elderly: can we do better? *Journal of the Royal Society of Medicine* 1994; **87**: 14–16.

9 Spagnoli A, Ostino G, Borga AD, *et al.* Drug compliance and unreported drugs in the elderly. *Journal of the American Geriatricians Society* 1989; **37**(7): 619–24.

10 Lorenc L & Braithwaite A Are older adults less compliant with prescribed medication than younger adults? *British Journal of Clinical Psychology* 1993; **32**(4): 485–92.

11 Cochrane RA, Mandal AR, Ledger-Scott M, *et al.* Changes in drug treatment after discharge from hospital in geriatric patients. *British Medical Journal* 1992; **305**(6855): 694–6.

12 Britten N, Brant S, Cairns A, *et al.* Continued prescribing of inappropriate drugs in general practice. *Journal of Clinical Pharmacology and Therapeutics* 1995; **20**(4): 199–205.

13 Haayer F Rational prescribing and sources of information. *Social Science and Medicine* 1982; **16**(23): 2017–23.

14 Strikwerda P, Bootsma-de Langeri AM, Berghuis F, *et al.* Drug therapy in a nursing home: favourable effect of feedback by the pharmacist on family physicians' prescribing behaviour. *Nederlands Tijdschrift voor Geneeskunde* 1994; **138**(35): 1770–4.

15 Anderson CM, Chambers S, Clamp M, *et al.* Can audit improve patient care? Effects of studying use of digoxin in general practice *British Medical Journal* 1988; **297**: 113–14.

16 Freer CB Study of medicine prescribing for elderly patients. *British Medical Journal* 1985; **290**(6475): 1113–15.

17 Cartwright A Collecting data about drug use by elderly people. *Pharm. Weekblad* 1990; **12**(2): 60–5.

18 Tamblyn RM, McLeod PJ, Abrahamowicz M, *et al.* Do too many cooks spoil the broth? Multiple physician involvement in the medical management of elder patients and potentially inappropriate drug combinations. *Canadian Medical Association Journal* 1996; **154**(8) 1177–84.

19 Ibanez Perez F & Olaskoaga Arrate A Prescription of cerebral and peripheral vasodilators in primary health care. *Atencion Primaria* 1994; **14**(3): 665–70.

20 Knox JDE Prescribing for the elderly in general practice: a review of current literature. *Journal of the Royal College of General Practitioners* 1980; **30** (1).

21 Cartwright A & Smith C *Elderly people: their medicines and their doctors.* Routledge, London 1988.

22 Iliffe S, Gallivan S, Haines A P, *et al.* Assessment of elderly people in general practice. 1: social circumstances and mental state. *British Journal of General Practice* 1991; **41**: 9–12.

23 Williamson J & Chopin JM Adverse reactions to prescribed drugs in the elderly: a multicentre investigation. *Age & Ageing* 1980; **9**: 73–80.

24 Bowman C & Morris J *Community institutional health care – emergence from refugee status.* Paper presented to the Royal Society of Medicine, Section of Geriatrics & Gerontology, March 23rd 1998.

25 Anonymous Elderly people: their medicines and their doctors *Drug & Therapeutic Bulletin* 1990; **28**(20): 77–9.

26 Bloom JA, Frank JW, Shafir MS, *et al.* Potentially undesirable prescribing and drug use among the elderly. *Canadian Family Physicians* 1993; **39**: 2337–45.

27 Burns E, Austin CA, & Bax NDS Elderly patients' understanding of their drug therapy: the effect of cognitive function. *Age & Ageing* 1990; **19**: 236–40.

28 Burns JMA, Sneddon I, Lovell M, *et al.* Elderly patients and their medication: a post-discharge follow-up study. *Age & Ageing* 1992; **21**: 178–81.

29 Shulman J, Shulman S, & Haines AP The prevention of adverse drug reactions – a potential role for pharmacists in the primary care team? *Journal of the Royal College of General Practioners* 1981; **31**(228): 429–34.

30 Walma EP, Hoes AW, Prins A, *et al.* Withdrawing long-term diuretic therapy in the elderly. *Family Medicine* 1993; **25**(10): 661–4.

31 Rhodes KE Prescription of diuretic drugs and monitoring of long-term use in one general practice. *British Journal of General Practice* 1992; **42**(355): 68–70.

32 Petri M, Bryant R, & Cumber P Thiazide treatment in elderly patients: the metabolic cost . *British Medical Journal* 1985; **291**: 1616.

33 Baldwin RC Late-life depression: undertreated? *British Medical Journal* 1988; **296**: 519.

34 Baldwin RC & Jolley DJ The prognosis of depression in old age *British Journal of Psychiatry* 1986; **149**: 574–83.

35 Moxley D *The Practice of Case Management* Sage, New York 1989.

36 Goodwin DR Nursing case management activities. *Journal of Nursing Administration* 1994; **24**(2): 29–34.

37 Pacala JT, Boult C, Hepburn KW, *et al* . Case management of older adults in health maintenance organizations. *Journal of American Geriatrics Society* 1995; **43**: 538–42.

38 Challis D & Davies B *Case management in community care.* Gower, Aldershot 1986

39 Stuck AE, Aronow HU, Steiner A, *et al.* A trial of annual, in-home, comprehensive geriatric assessments for elderly people living in the community. *New England Journal of Medicine* 1995; **333**: 1184–9.

40 Grimshaw JM & Russell IT Effect of clinical guidelines on medical practice: a systematic review of rigorous evaluations. *Lancet* 1993; **342**: 1317–22.

41 Freemantle N, Harvey EL, Wolf F, *et al.* Printed educational materials to improve the behaviour of health care professionals and patient outcomes. *Cochrane Library* (updated 28 Feb 1997), Issue 1, 1998.

42 Implementing clinical practice guidelines: can guidelines be used to improve clinical practice? *Effective Health Care Bulletin No. 8* University of Leeds, Leeds 1994.

43 Bugeja G, Kumar A & Banerjee AK Exclusion of elderly people from clinical research: a descriptive study of published reports.*British Medical Journal* 1997; **315**: 1059.

44 Avorn J Including elderly people in clinical trials. *British Medical Journal* 1997; **315**: 1033–4.

45 Townsend J, McKinnon M, Machen I, *et al. Evidence-based guidelines for older people in primary care.* WONCA/EGPRW Conference, Majorca, May 22-24th 1999.

46 Knottnerus JA & Dinant GJ Medicine- based evidence, a prerequisite for evidence -based medicine. *British Medical Journal* 1997; **315**: 1109–10.

47 Dickie S *Evaluation of the 75-and-over checks: report 3. The social services/primary care interface.* Dept of Primary Care, UCLMS, London 1996.

48 Morris R Community care and the fundholder. *British Medical Journal* 1993; **306**: 635–7.

49 Maclister-Smith E Linkworking in Wiltshire: the health perspective. *Primary Care Management* 1994; **5**(9): 6–8.

50 Challis L & Pearson J *Report on the evaluation of linkworker pilots in Wiltshire* School of Social Work, University of Bath 1993.

51 Robinson B Lyme cordial. *Health Services Journal,* August 5th: 1993; 20–3.

52 Sheppard M Contact and collaboration with general practitioners: a comparison of social workers and community psychiatric nurses. *British Journal of Social Work* 1992; **22**: 419–36.

53 Corney RH Factors affecting the operation and success of social work attachment schemes to general practice. *Journal of the Royal College of general Practitioners* 1980; **30**: 149–58.

54 McKinstry B Successful liaison between the health team and social workers in

Blackburn, West Lothian. *British Medical Journal* 1987; **294**: 221–2.

55 Ross F & Tissier J The care management interface with general practice: a case study. *Health and Social Care in the Community* 1997; **5** (3): 153–61.

56 Wistow G Collaboration between health and local authorities: why is it necessary? *Social Policy & administration* 1982; **16**: 44–62.

57 lliffe S, Eden A, Downs M, *et al.* The diagnosis and management of dementia in primary care: development, implementation and evaluation of a national training programme. *Ageing & Mental Health* 1999; **3**(2): 129–35.

58 Excerpta Medica *Action in Alzheimer's training day delegates record book.* Excerpta Medica, Oxford 1997.

59 Linstone HA & Turoff M *The Delphi method: techniques and applications.* Addison-Wesley, Boston, Massachusetts 1975.

60 White E A Delphi study on psychiatric nursing. *Nursing Times* 1991; **87**: 48–9.

61 Bond S & Bond J A Delphi survey of clinical nursing research priorities. *Journal of Advanced Nursing* 1982; **7**: 565–75.

62 Knowles MS *Androgogy in action: applying modern principles of adult learning* Jossey Bass, San Francisco 1984.

63 Brown A Independent learning. In Henry H, Byrne K, & Engel C (eds) *Imperatives in medical education: the Newcastle approach.* University of Newcastle, Australia 1997.

64 World Health Organization *Learning to work together for health: the team approach* WHO Technical Report Services 1988.

65 Lorenz RA & Pichert JW Impact of interprofessional training on medical students' willingness to accept clinical responsibility. *Medicine and Education* 1986; **20**: 195–200.

66 Eccles M, Clarke J, Livingstone M, *et al.* North of England evidence-based guidelines development project: summary version of the evidence-based guidelines for primary care management of dementia. *British Medical Journal* 1998; **317**: 802–8.

67 Alzheimer's Disease Society *Dementia in the community: a management plan for general practice* Alzheimer's Disease Society, London 1994.

68 Downs M The role of general practice and the primary care team in dementia diagnosis and management. *Int. J. Geriat. Psych.* 1996; **11**: 937–42.

CHAPTER FOUR

Establishing the infrastructure for quality health care

This chapter considers the elements in the organization of primary health care which significantly contribute to the quality of health care. We will argue that organizational and professional cultures play a significant role in the way that health and social care is delivered. Attention to recognizing the current differences will assist in developing a culture of integrated working which gives the prime focus to the older person rather than individual professional roles. The chapter considers issues in collaboration and teamworking, communication and networking, and team effectiveness and quality.

The impetus for collaboration and teamwork

Primary health care for older people includes treatment of illness, promotion of health, rehabilitation, management and care in chronic conditions, as well as care and symptom control in those dying. All of these endeavours take place against a backdrop of social and demographic changes, economic constraints in public spending, and public policy that emphasizes intersectoral collaboration in the provision of care. Primary health care professionals repeatedly describe their work environments as one of increasing workload against dwindling resources with greater specification being placed on them by central government(s) and a more demanding public.

Collaboration and teamwork have long been advocated [1,2] as a means of providing effective primary health care. However, there is an equally long history of critiquing the reality of teamwork in primary health care.[3,4] Many commentators have pointed to employment status differences, professional cultural differences, geographical separation, and membership of multiple teams as real barriers.[5–7]

The 1990s have witnessed shifts which give new impetus to collaboration and teamworking. Three of these are discussed below:

- legislation for collaboration
- general practice organizational development
- role shifts

Collaboration has been enshrined in legislation in a way markedly different to previous decades. The NHS and Community Care Act 1990[8] legislates for collaboration in planning and delivering individuals' care as well as service planning. This has been reinforced by the establishment of primary care groups[9] based on collaboration between general practices as well as between professionals in the planning, provision, and monitoring of health care services for small populations. The Primary Care Act Pilots[10] allow for financial collaboration between previously separate funding streams of general medical services (GMS) and hospital and community health services (HCHS) to provide integrated services. Similar possibilities are being mooted between the funding streams of local authorities and health authorities, bringing down the 'Berlin Wall'[11] between 'health' and 'social' care.

Developments in the organization of, and demands on, general practice during the nineties provided a more fertile environment for an increase in collaboration and teamwork. The 1990 GP contract requirements, together with the administration of fundholding, led to the phenomenal growth in the direct employment of administrative staff and nurses in general practice.[12] The emergence of the general practice as a powerful unit in purchasing and/or commissioning health services influenced closer working arrangements between community nurses and practices , including experiments with integrated nursing teams.[13,14] A new level of collaboration between practices was evidenced in the establishment of multifunds and out-of-hours collectives.

The shift in delivery of certain types of care from secondary to primary care has necessitated more collaborative working between the sectors, for example the developments of Hospital at Home schemes and intermediate care schemes. This shift is also one of the changes which has made primary health care professionals redefine role boundaries. The most obvious is the shift in roles from general practitioners to practice nurses and nurse practitioners.[15]

Why collaborate and with whom?

Despite the invocations to work in multidisciplinary teams there appears to be little direct evidence of the benefits to patients in primary care,[16] but from other domains there is evidence of more efficient health care delivery and increased staff motivation.[17] An intuitive list of the benefits of collaborative working would include factors such as:

- care given by a group is greater than that given by one
- rare skills and knowledge are used more appropriately
- duplication and gaps in care-giving and other activities are avoided
- peer influence and informal learning raises standards of care
- team members have greater job satisfaction and are better able to cope with stress
- potential for more creative and lateral solutions to problems.

Many descriptions of primary health care teams are mere lists of potential professionals and people from the voluntary sector who might form part of a team. It is a term which is widely used and its frequent use obscures the fact that it is being used to describe different functional groupings and collaborative acts 'rather than a single monolithic team'.[18] The Royal College of General Practitioners (RCGP)[19] has argued that there is a core primary care team of GPs and employees of the practice surrounded by a wider multiprofessional network. However, there is also a distinction to be made between the members of the team who are partners in the financial business of the practice, those who are directly employed by the GPs, and those who are collaborators in the provision of health and social care for some or all of the practice population. To ignore this distinction means ignoring one of the biggest potential sources of tension in this entity called a primary health care team.

Creating a climate for teamworking

'A team is a group of people who make different contributions towards the achievement of a common goal.'[20]

The essential characteristics of teamwork can be summarized as:

- each member of the team having a clear understanding of their own functions and understanding the contribution of others, recognizing common interests and skills, in the achievement of the common goal
- the team works by pooling knowledge skills and resources
- all members share the responsibility for the outcome of their decisions
- the effectiveness of the team is related to its capability to carry out its work and manage itself as an interdependent group of people.

By focusing on a definition of a team and some core characteristics, it is obvious that teams or work groups with different membership will form at different times in the pursuit of specific common goals. Commentators on organizational development place the explicit sharing of purpose, values, and culture as essential to effective team functioning.[21] They also argue that where there are clear team goals with built-in performance feedback, the team effectiveness improves. This point will be returned to later.

The Adelaide Medical Centre primary health care team offers a rare published example of becoming explicit in writing as to their purpose, with annual objectives for subgroups to work together to achieve.[22] This is detailed in Box 4.1. This example demonstrates a team with a specific identify, collaborating and planning at an organizational level.

The purpose and goals are the concerns of the entire team and focus is on the whole practice population. Increasingly, practices have strategic service plans and annual business plans – either as a result of fundholding or as a requirement of the health authority – which should detail annual objectives and goals. The extent to which these type of plans are developed collaboratively or even shared beyond the practice principals depends on the level of teamworking in that practice.

Box 4.1 *Extracts from the Adelaide Medical Centre primary health care team manifesto*[22]

Aims

- To provide an exemplary primary health care service for patients registered with the practice.
- To work together as a team.
- To educate ourselves, our patients, our colleagues, trainees, and students from any discipline.

43 objectives follow, detailing: acute care, prescribing, women's health, health promotion and preventative care, chronic care, terminal care, patient relations, teamwork, teaching, and audit and information systems.

The following are examples of objectives:
'2.8 Patients on long-term medication will be reviewed at least annually.
4.5 All patients over 75 will be functionally assessed annually.
6.2 Bereaved relatives will be visited soon after a death.
7.2 The team will endeavour to maintain contact with, or visit, hospitalized patients.
8.4 All team members will have ease of access to each other and be respected as an integral part of the whole.
10.2 Manual registers will be maintained for births, deaths, malignant disease, minor surgical operations, and dangerous drugs.'

The team includes a practice nurse, district nurses, community psychiatric nurse, community midwife, practice manager, receptionist, secretaries, health visitor, and GPs.

Health professionals are more familiar with objectives linked to a specific patient's care or treatment. This patient-level teamworking has been called the intrinsic team.[23] Here the goals may range from cure to care, for example:

- supporting a patient to die in the place of their choice with pain and discomfort minimized
- to provide rehabilitation to independent living, post hip replacement
- to heal a venous leg ulcer within 14 weeks.

Between the organizational and the patient level is teamworking on objectives for a specific function either of the organization or the team. Examples of this include:

- to provide a chronic disease management clinic
- to provide home visits
- to provide an out-of-hours service.

Leadership is important for all teams. Leadership styles that contribute to collaboratively working will be facilitative rather than didactic. Authoritarian styles of leadership are unlikely to use the skills and knowledge of all the collaborators appropriately, unlikely to develop collective responsibility, and unlikely to develop a creative working atmosphere.[24] Examining the three levels of teamworking above, it is obvious that the leadership role could be taken by different people at different times.

Physical proximity, social proximity, and positive motivation are prerequisites to collaboration and teamworking, as is interaction between members.[25] Therefore size of membership is an important factor, with three to six offered as the most effective group size for decision-making and communicating.[26] These become real issues for those professionals who are required to work in close collaboration but who are not based together, and who may be required to function in larger groupings, such as primary care groups. Repeated studies from the 1960s onwards have shown that collaboration is closest between GPs and district nurses and health visitors when the nurses are physically based in the same building and are attached to no more than two general practices.[27] Recent studies of joint working between social work staff and primary care staff support the value of close physical proximity.[28]

A number of sliding scales have been developed to describe the level of collaborative work in primary care teamwork.[29] These range from complete isolation where clinical information, referral, or requests are passed between doctors, nurses, and social workers via administrative staff or relatives, so that the professionals never talk or meet. At the other end of the scale they describe full collaboration where professionals' work is fully integrated with each other. Three levels of teamworking have been described:[30]

- nominal – isolated working
- convenient – tasks by hierarchical delegation
- committed – fully integrated working.

Table 4.1 is a model for primary care practitioners to assess their level of collaborative working.[31]

Conflict in teams

Paradoxically, while teamwork can contribute to high levels of job satisfaction, it can also be a source of stress for individuals. Teamwork can expose role ambiguity and opposing values. It is, however, interpersonal conflict which can lead to the most intractable stress for individual members.[32] In primary care, the multiple professional groupings add particular dimensions for interpersonal conflict and it would be naïve to underestimate this. So not only are there possibilities for conflict within one group – for example the partners in the practice – but also between groups, such as the practice nurses, district nurses, and health visitors, who are all technically community nurses. Huntington[33] has provided a useful model for understanding the underlying causes of tension in primary health care teams. She argued that conflict could be seen as the interplay between three elements: identity, territory, and control (Figure 4.1).

Table 4.1 *Assessment of levels of collaboration (from Pritchard 1995)*[31]

Cooperation in:	Nominal team	Convenient team	Committed team
Team goal-setting	no explicit goals	follow doctors orders	shared explicit goals
Role perceptions	stereotypes common	some understanding	roles clearly understood
Professional status	wide differences	differences inhibit cooperation	differences ignored
Referral of patients	to the agency not the individual	referral by delegation	easy two-way
Interaction within team	minimal	some	close regular, formal,and informal
Mutual trust	lacking	guarded	strong and developing
Communication	frequent	sometimes	exceptional failures
Confidentiality	a problem	problems partly solved	not a problem
Preventative care	not possible	possible	optimum conditions
Advice to patients	inconsistent	poor coordination	consistent

Each of these elements are important to every individual in order to have a personal sense of worth and commitment to the team objectives. An infringement of one element affects another. Many issues of conflict over seemingly trivial issues become more understandable if analysed in this framework – Box 4.2 gives one such analysis. While such incidents may seem small they often contribute to the overall climate of teamworking. Multiple small areas of tension build to significant non-cooperation between individuals. A leadership role which allows these types of issues to be discussed and

Figure 4.1 *Conflict can be seen as the interplay between three elements – identity, territory, and control.*[33]

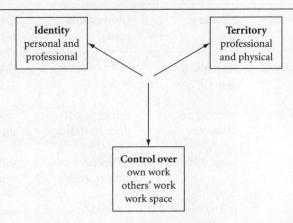

Box 4.2 *Case example*

'The doctors barge in without knocking on our work – they wouldn't accept that if we did it to them' (practice nurse)[34]

This issue for the practice nurse can be interpreted as:

- the nurses cannot control access to their workspace
- the nurses cannot protect their professional consultation with patients
- the nurses cannot protect the patients' privacy
- the nurses' professional status is of a low level that does not require the common courtesy of knocking prior to entry.

Each element of control, territory, and identity is infringed by a seemingly small omission in behaviour by the GPs.

---

negotiated can change the culture of working practices. Sometimes the resolution of serious conflict may need a neutral outside person to help.

Team-building

The last 15 years have seen a wide range of initiatives to support team-building and development in primary care. Many of these have used facilitators funded by the health authority or through specific project grants. Some facilitators have focused explicitly on team-building, such as the health education authorities primary health care team workshops for health promotion,[35] while others have used team-building as an integral part of a specific project such as the introduction of total quality management to general practice,[36] community-orientated primary care pilots,[37] or an overall primary care development project such as the London Implementation Zone Initiatives[38] or Team Care Valleys.[39] Some commentators argue that facilitated workshops or away days on team-building have inherent problems. These include difficulties if only part of the team are released for the event and problems in sustaining the momentum and enthusiasm generated by the event when faced by the normal work environment. These type of problems have led others to argue that the most effective team-building work appears to take place when there is a clear, practice-based project to be undertaken.[40]

Sources of information on team-building in primary care include:

- Wilson A *Changing practices in primary care: a facilitators handbook.* Health Education Authority, London 1994.
- Munro K *Teamworking in Practice.* Radcliffe Medical Press, Oxford 1991.
- Pritchard. P & Pritchard J *Teamwork for primary and shared care: a practical workbook* (2nd Edition). Oxford University Press, Oxford 1995.

Communication

It is self-evident that communication is crucial to high-quality care. Where there is little collaboration between professionals in primary care, communication failures are frequent. Public enquiries into fatalities, health ombudsman reports, and summaries of patients' complaints, repeatedly point to a failure in communication whether through written records between professionals, through information not being passed from one professional to another, or failure to communicate adequately and appropriately with the patient and carers.

The following case study illustrates the effect on care for an older person when there are multiple communication failures.

Mrs K. was 86 years old. She played bridge regularly three times a week, taking a taxi to friends' homes when they did not visit her. Underweight, with a body mass index (BMI) of 17, she ate little but described at length how she had always had a 'nervous' stomach, and politely declined any advice, further investigation, or medication. With the assistance of a cleaner she kept her large flat in order, and her nephew (who lived 70 miles away) visited once a week and did her shopping. Her flat was above street level, and her front door was approached by a steep flight of steps which caused her and her neighbours some anxiety when she slowly ascended and descended them.

After one bridge party she decided to stop the taxi on the way home and go to the bank. She slipped on the pavement and fell hard, but refused any help other than being restored to her feet and put back in her cab. The driver took her home and helped her up the steps to her door, but with great difficulty. A neighbour, about 10 years younger than her, helped her into her flat and, realizing that she was in considerable pain, called her GP.

Her GP visited before the evening surgery and found her shaken but not seriously injured. She had no signs of a femoral fracture, was able to weight-bear, and could shuffle around her flat – just. She was determined to stay at home and categorically refused admission to hospital, even to the GP ward where her own doctor could organize her care. It was obvious to her GP that she would need some extra help at home, in the short term, so she telephoned the social services 'one-stop shop' to request an urgent assessment of need, and arranged to revist the next day, at the same time.

Next morning Mrs K.'s nephew telephoned the surgery to ask what was being done, and the plan was explained. He commented that no contact from social services had occurred, and called back later to say that he was taking his aunt to his home, and that the visit planned was no longer necessary.

A week later he wrote to the GP complaining about the standard of care given, saying that Mrs K. had needed admission to a nursing home, that she had suffered a pelvic fracture, and that she should not have been left alone overnight on the day of the accident. Mrs K.'s nephew suggested that the practice might pay for the nursing home placement.

He also complained in writing to the Director of Social Services who could find no record of the request for help being made from the GP.

A meeting between the GP and Mrs K.'s nephew resolved the conflict. The nephew accepted that the GP's actions had not been in error, that his aunt's resolute independence had to be respected, and that the decision to transfer her from her home to a nursing home had been his alone. Nevertheless, he pressed the point about the failed communication between the GP and social services, and asked for action to be taken on this.

A subsequent meeting between the GP and the local social service manager clarified the lines of communication and the likely response times of services to urgent requests.

Any attempt to improve communications needs to address the barriers both at an individual practitioner level and at an organizational level. Below is a list of some key barriers to communication between patients, professionals, and service providers:

- lack of understanding of the scope of individual roles
- lack of comprehension of the system or service (for example, the community care assessment process)
- lack of understanding of how individual professional roles contribute to accessing or negotiating for other services on behalf of the patient
- lack of systems to inform other relevant professionals of activities carried out for a shared patient
- lack of opportunities to develop personal contact with the other care providers
- the use of jargon and technical terms by professionals
- physical problems such as visual or hearing loss
- anxiety or fear at the time of consultation
- cultural, social class, language, and gender differences.

It's good to talk – trite but true!

The most effective method of communication, whether sharing information on patients, making decisions, or getting to know a new colleague, is by talking to each other. This effectiveness is increased by supporting written information – whether that's the person's telephone extension number or details of a patient referral. However, different professional cultures place different interpretations on ways of talking to each other. These result in a range of stereotypes for professional behaviours such as GPs who are allergic to meetings while other groups such as social workers and psychiatric nurses are perceived as doing little else but sitting in meetings. The work practices of different groups often lend themselves to these stereotypes, for example 'the doctors only talk to us district nurses in the corridor.'[41] The reality is that time is precious. All professionals balance the benefits from meetings against the time cost in deciding whether, how often, and when to meet.

In their favour, meetings offer the chance:

- to interact with others to form a team
- to share with others – whether that's workload, anxieties about a particular patient, skills, or bright ideas
- for different perspectives and knowledge to be offered on identifying and creatively solving problems
- for different opinions and views to be verbalized and explored
- of protected time to reflect on an issue and plan for the future.

The productivity of meetings is directly related to having:

- a clear purpose, with an agreed time span and frequency linked to the purpose
- an agenda which lists the items, the activity for the meeting, and the lead contributor for that item, e.g. (1) review of Mrs Brown's care – Dr Jones (2) new diabetic care protocol for agreement – Nurse Green (3) Agree date of next meeting – all
- the appropriate people for the purpose of the meeting
- a chairperson who is clear on his/her role
- someone who takes notes of decisions and is responsible for circulating them (including to absentees).

The case management process outlined in Chapter 3 depends upon this kind of structured approach. Good practice would indicate that any regular meetings should be reviewed at least annually by the participants to decide whether that meeting can cease or the productivity be improved through a different format or through invitation of others.

Networking

Another type of dialogue that is vital in the primary health care of older people is networking. Networking refers to a process of getting to know and getting known to other people in the complex mosaic of health, local authority, independent, and voluntary sector provision in any area. At the most basic level it can be introducing yourself and putting 'a name and a face/voice together'. The real trick of networking for the benefit of a patient group as opposed to individual professional development is to begin to make contacts outside one's own professional grouping or service. The benefits include:

- a wider knowledge of what is available to the older person
- a level of personal contact that makes it easier to seek another person's opinion or make a referral
- the potential to collaborate in innovative or creative ways.

Single-discipline networking tends to happen through continuing educational events such as seminars led by consultants, specialist nurses, or social workers. Multidisciplinary education and learning tends to be the exception and therefore the opportunity to network may be lost. Primary care groups should seriously consider their role in promoting multiprofessional continuing education. Multidisciplinary networking beneficial to older people is often promoted around an issue such as 'cold weather planning' in a particular area, led by the local authority. In some communities there may be a forum which brings older people and anyone involved in providing care to come together informally, to meet and to learn from each other. This type of gathering has in the past been developed by concerned professionals such as GPs, health visitors, and social workers or from the voluntary sector such as voluntary councils, religious leaders, and community development workers. This aspect of networking will be discussed again in Chapter 12.

The promise of electronic communication

Even if we have an ambition to know and work closely with everyone concerned with the health care of older people, the organizational complexities of the tasks demand administrative systems that assist communication and speedy, confidential transfer of information.

Information technology is beginning to offer a range of options to improve communication to this wide community network such as e-mail, links between computer systems, and intranets. The NHS Information Technology Strategy[42] provides an exciting policy backdrop to exploiting information technology for the benefit of patient care. Box 4.3 lists some of the 15 specific targets; of these, four are specifically centred on general practice.

The new NHS Information Technology Strategy has placed the electronic health record in primary care as its building block for the 21st century – a 'first generation of person-based electronic health records, providing the basis of lifelong core clinical information and electronic transfer of patient records between GPs'. The vision for this record is that it holds subsets of core information from secondary care, community health services, mental health services, and social care records and thus supports integrated care. For many people involved in providing health care to older people this offers a solution to the problem of multiple professional records held in isolation, for others it raises concerns of confidentiality and security of information.

The current reality for the older patient and their carers is having to repeat information to each professional and service they meet and a sense of frustration at the inability of one sector to know what the other is doing. At the moment about 85% of all practices have patient records on computer. However, there are a variety of software systems in use with no common,

---

Box 4.3 *Targets from the NHS Information Technology Strategy*[42]

- Reaching agreement with the professions on the security of electronic systems and networks carrying patient-identifiable clinical information.
- Developing and implementing a first generation of person-based electronic health records, providing the basis of lifelong core clinical information with electronic transfer of patient records between GPs.
- Implementing comprehensive integrated clinical systems to support the joint needs of GPs and the extended primary care team.
- Ensuring that all acute hospitals have the ability to undertake all patient administration and are capable of supporting clinical orders, results reporting, prescribing, and multiprofessional care pathways.
- Connecting all computerized GP practices to the NHS net.
- Providing 24-hour emergency care access to relevant information from patient records.
- Using the NHS net for appointment booking, referrals, discharge information, radiology, and laboratory requests and results.
- Community prescribing with electronic links to GPs and the Prescription Pricing Authority.
- Opening a National Electronic Library for Health with accredited clinical reference material on the NHS net.

---

agreed patient-record structure. The sole use of electronic records by GPs is at present a breach of contract.[43] Likewise, staff from trusts or local authorities attached to the practice are usually required to use completely different computerized systems for recording their patient contacts and invariably use paper records as well. Figure 4.2 illustrates the number of unconnected records held by different services and professionals on one older person with a range of problems and a high level of dependency on health and social services.

While general practice has been coming to grips with computerization, staff in community trusts have been using computerized records in the main for administrative purposes, duplicating their records from the patient/client paper notes. The advent of the internal market made the demands for activity data more stringent. The experiences of most nursing staff of the electronic age has left many of them justifiably cynical. A cynicism borne out by the Audit Commission[44] which estimated that the community nurses and professionals allied to medicine spent the equivalent of a quarter of their time collecting data and dealing with it. They went further to put a figure on this of approximately six million pounds per annum on an average-size community trust – a figure that might interest any PCG member considering how to identify funding for changing local services for older people. Twelve months after the publication of this report, the new NHS Information Strategy stated there will be an urgent review of the time spent by community health staff in collecting data on activity for central government.[45]

While the utopia of a shared, integrated electronic record is being worked on, the more pragmatic approach is to develop systems which ensure exchange

Figure 4.2 Case example of multiple record keeping.

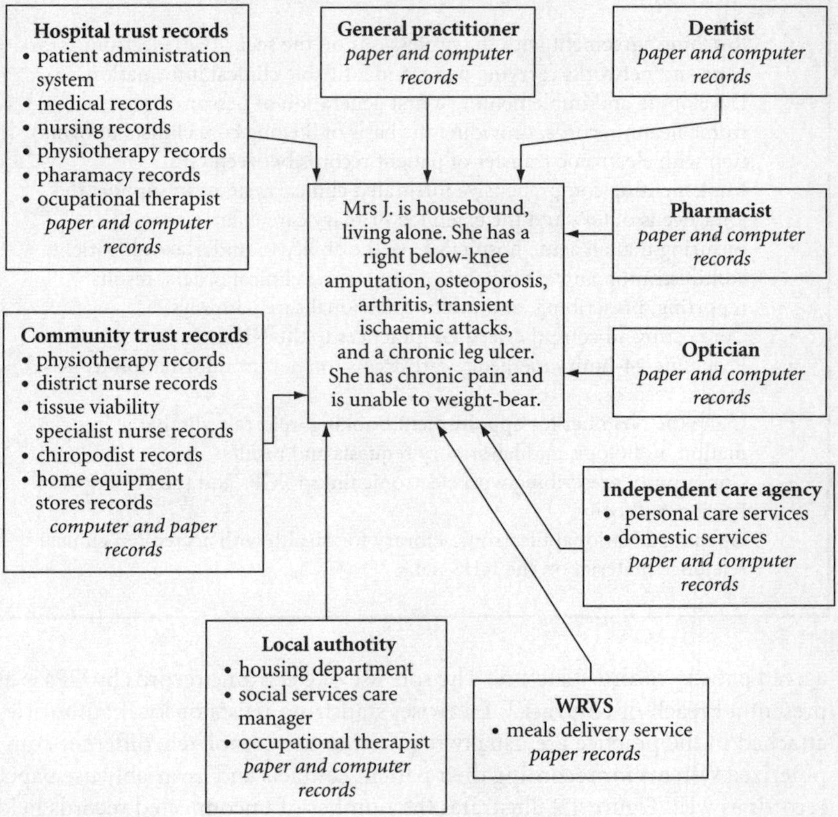

Hospital trust records
- patient administration system
- medical records
- nursing records
- physiotherapy records
- pharamacy records
- ocupational therapist
  paper and computer records

General practitioner
paper and computer records

Dentist
paper and computer records

Mrs J. is housebound, living alone. She has a right below-knee amputation, osteoporosis, arthritis, transient ischaemic attacks, and a chronic leg ulcer. She has chronic pain and is unable to weight-bear.

Pharmacist
paper and computer records

Community trust records
- physiotherapy records
- district nurse records
- tissue viability specialist nurse records
- chiropodist records
- home equipment stores records
  computer and paper records

Optician
paper and computer records

Independent care agency
- personal care services
- domestic services
  paper and computer records

Local authotity
- housing department
- social services care manager
- occupational therapist
  paper and computer records

WRVS
- meals delivery service
  paper records

of details on each professional's activity without creating another form-filing nightmare. Some examples of how this has been done include:

- agreed shared-care protocols between primary and secondary care on chronic disease management, supported by patient-held records
- giving district nurses and health visitors access to the practice patient record (unfortunately, in many areas this has not meant they could stop data entry in Trust systems, although now the NHS Information Strategy is finally acknowledging the futility of this duplication)
- patient-held health records, particularly for over-75 checks and in chronic disease management
- combined district nursing and local authority records held in the older person's home
- copies of the key community care documents stating needs and care plans given to the older person, as well as the GP and district nurse.

Developing effective communication is just one part of becoming an effective team or work group. One of the key elements stressed endlessly by commentators is that there is a method of feedback or review on the team performance – basically a way of saying how are we doing, are we doing what we set out do, can we improve? The next section goes on to consider systematic ways of answering these questions for a team.

Team effectiveness and the clinical governance agenda

If the common purpose of the team is to provide high-quality health promotion and care for older people then how does the team judge success? The challenge in primary health care is to become more explicit as to what constitutes quality health care for older people. The individual patient judges the quality of the encounter with doctor or nurse not just on their manner and actions taken but on the experience of trying to contact them, their treatment by reception staff, waiting times, and evidence of communication between different services involved. Older people with multiple health and social problems inevitably have more complicated treatment and care negotiated around the needs, desires, and abilities of the individual and their personal network. The more complex the health care the greater the volume of doctors, nurses, social workers, therapists, administrative staff, and family/friends involved in the care mosaic. Each person and profession will bring their perspective on the elements that constitute good-quality care, and often rank them differently.

'The concept of quality [in health care] is ambiguous: impossible to define but we know it when we see it.'[46]

At the bottom line, most teams would define their effectiveness in terms of achieving what they set out to do, irrespective of the team's organizational level. However, in caring for older people there is often not a clear end-point from which to judge outcomes from. In some instances, the complexity of the health and social problems combined with intricate networks of relationships means that a team may need to ask other questions beside 'did we achieve our objectives.' Most teams need to judge their performance using more than one dimension and from more than one perspective.

Two of the most widely known frameworks for examining quality of care are that proposed by Donabedian[47] and Maxwell.[48] Donabedian classified health care into three components of structure, process, and outcome. *Structure* of care describes all the resources, including environment and people, that combine to deliver the care. The *process* of care includes all the procedures, events, and interpersonal aspects. The *outcome* of care is change in the health status directly attributable to the structure and process of a health care intervention. These three components are helpful when examining success and quality in health care of older people.

Maxwell proposed that the following dimensions should be considered in judging any health care activity:

- *relevance (or appropriateness)* – the service is actually required by the individual or the population

- *effectiveness* – the extent to which a health care intervention achieves the desired outcome
- *efficiency* – resources are well used
- *acceptability* – reasonable expectations of the patient or community are met
- *accessibility* – structural access is within accepted norms
- *equity* – there is a fair share for all the community.

Maxwell argued that each element needed to be considered separately using different methods of assessment , subsequent to acceptable levels or standards being agreed. He went on to develop this into a framework[49] incorporating Donobedian's ideas. Using a case study, we have used the framework to explore how a wider set of questions might be posed beyond examining progress against objectives or a care plan.

Mrs P. is 75 years old, originally from Lithuania, and speaks little English. She lives with a mobile but frail sister who translates – her husband having died three years ago. Her daughter lives 30 miles away and is a working mother with a young family. The sisters have close connections with the Lithuanian church community. She is a diabetic, dependent on insulin. Her recent second stroke has left her with very limited mobility, impaired her speech, and removed her gag reflex. She has a gastrostomy. She has control of her bladder and bowels but is occasionally incontinent, unable to wait until two carers arrive to assist her onto the commode. She was discharged home three months after admission, with a care package, following a comprehensive needs assessment by the hospital social work care manager. Home carers visit three times a day to provide personal hygiene services and help Mrs P. get up and return to bed. The district nursing service visits twice a day to give the insulin, gastrostomy feeds, as well as monitor blood sugars and her general health. Her GP has known her and her family for over 20 years. She visits her on return from hospital and subsequently to review medication as well as assess her emotional state as she is extremely tearful. The gastrostomy feed and other supplies are delivered directly to the home by the commercial suppliers. The frail sister has not had a carer's assessment of need undertaken as the case is awaiting assignment to a community social work care manager. This sister recently consulted the GP in the surgery about her own distress, fears, and difficulties in coping. The GP and the district nurse meet to review their care treatment, and plans.

Their initial care objectives included:

- to enable Mrs P. to return home
- to provide personal hygiene and care services
- to continue the process of rehabilitation to maximum possible independence
- to treat her diabetes with insulin and monitor in accordance with their protocols
- to maintain the gastrostomy and provide nutrition via it
- to provide support to her sister in her role as carer.

In their review, pooling their information, they conclude:

- yes they have managed some of these objectives, e.g. she is at home
- some objectives are ongoing, e.g. providing personal care

- some objectives need a new approach to improve how they are doing e.g. the rehabilitation work
- new problems and issues have presented themselves which they need to address, e.g. the sister's distress and burden as a carer, and Mrs P.'s emotional health.

Table 4.2 indicates how the type of quality framework outlined above might widen the scope of the questions to be asked in reviewing how the team was doing in this case.

These questions begin to reveal that the information for judging the team performance may come from sources other than the professional perspective – a point we will return to later in this chapter.

Integral to any review is the commitment to act on the findings. Identifying the actions needed, deciding who will do what, and by when are important parts of the process as is setting the next joint review date. From this case study there would be a range of answers and action points. High on the list would be contacting the area community care team manager in order to get a named community-based social worker or care manager working with these sisters, the GP, and the district nurse.

Team effectiveness at a functional and organizational level

The question for the team operating at a functional or organizational level is 'how are we doing with this *group* of patients?'. At this point the team needs a more systematic infrastructure to help answer the questions posed in such a framework described above. However, just as at the intrinsic team level there needs to be a commitment to action. All of the theoretical models for improving quality involve a cyclical (or hopefully more a spiral) process. This includes focused activities such as clinical audit or whole systems such as total quality management (TQM) or continuous quality improvement (CQI). This cycle includes the following elements:

(1) identifying a topic or issue
(2) agreeing and stating criteria, processes, and standards
(3) publicizing, implementing, adopting, or teaching about them
(4) documenting the care, process, and service
(5) comparing it with the stated standards in point 2 – and in some instances with other teams' performances as well
(6) identifying areas for improvement or change
(7) planning for that change
(8) moving back round into the cycle again at point 2 or 3, amended now to become 2a or 3a.

The nineties saw the widespread development of clinical and service criteria on which to judge health care and social care. The reforms of the early nineties brought into being for the first time:

Table 4.2 *A framework for considering the quality of care in the case of Mrs P.*

	Structure	Process	Outcome
Effectiveness	Have we used a comprehensive initial assessment of health and social issues and problems? Do we have the right staff with the right skills providing the care? Do we have the right equipment in the home?	Are we offering the most effective care and treatment for *all* the conditions? Have we identified all the health and social issues/problems whose interplay might impact on effectiveness?	Have we achieved the level of health status we set out to achieve in this time period? Is what we are doing making a difference?
Efficiency	Are we avoiding extravagance in equipment, suppliers, medication, and staffing?	Is there any duplication of activity between ourselves? Have we left gaps in the care? Are we promoting continuity of care, carers, and advice rather than fragmentation?	
Appropriateness	Is care within the home the most appropriate venue for all concerned?		Have we asked the patient and her relatives their opinions of the care and treatment to date?

Acceptability
Are we providing the care in ways that are acceptable to the sisters? Have we explained adequately our activities and plans to them and the rest of the family?

When they have tried to contact people in each service or attend appointments, have they been able to?

Access
Are we sure Mrs P. has been able to understand and communicate with us in a way that is not affected by her sister's relationship? Have we ensured these sisters have the contact details and understand how to contact each service?

Equity
Is this person being offered the same level of support as any other in a similar position of need?

Have we ensured that despite Mrs P. having English as a second language she has been able to participate fully in the decision-making on the care and treatment given to her?

- a culture of patients' or users' rights
- a policy commitment to audit, particularly medical audit
- quality specification and monitoring processes within the plethora of contracts and service level agreements made between health authorities, general practices and provider trusts. This also included the contract with GPs where targets in screening, health promotion, and preventative activities attracted financial reimbursement.

During this period many systematic methods of judging quality were developed, including the use of independent external review such as the King's Fund Primary Care Organizational Audit Scheme, British Standards Institute ISO 9000, and national schemes for benchmarking.

The central policy initiatives on quality over the last 10 years reflect Maxwell's framework, culminating in the present administration's bold initiative of a new national framework for assessing performance. This focuses on:

- health improvement
- fair access to services
- effective delivery of health care
- efficiency
- patient and carer experience
- health outcomes of NHS care.

These areas are mirrored in the social services performance assessment framework and the Best Value regime.[51] The present administration has developed all of these elements and charged primary care groups with the corporate responsibility of 'clinical governance'.[52] Each PCG has lead members identified to take forward clinical governance and quality development across the whole PCG in accordance with the national guidance.[53] The suggestions in the policy guidance for the tasks are:

- defining information fields to carry out audits and reviews (including standards to measure quality and measure changes in performance)
- agreeing clinical audits (which may cross service boundaries) with participants
- ensuring action is taken to improve care, knowledge, skills, and attitudes.[54]

The underlying principles of clinical governance are based on planned quality assurance and risk management programmes linked to staff and organizational development.

We would argue that a team needs to agree in advance in what ways it is going to have feedback and judge its performance. Within trusts and social services this is standard practice at an organizational level. Many practices do this in their annual plans, while others may wish to consider the advantages of annual clinical governance plans. These:

- allow an explicit process for deciding what are the important areas to have feedback about – rather than one person's particular passion

- allow a planned approach to providing feedback on any developments or changes the team has been working on
- make the team look realistically at what is achievable within the available resources rather than create a wish list
- provide ownership and a commitment to take the process seriously as part of both the practice and the wider team.

We will now consider some specific techniques in judging performance.

Examining clinical quality

During the nineties, primary care professionals are most likely to have been exposed to clinical audit as a method of judging quality, although there have been other initiatives to which we will return. By 1995 it was estimated that 86% of practices were involved in at least one audit activity.[55] A major impetus came from the establishment of medical audit advisory groups, with the funding for audit officers to aid and support practices. As the decade progressed it became clearer that the term 'clinical audit' more clearly reflected the nature of multidisciplinary health care, and this was promoted through all the policy and funding initiatives. The membership of these groups widened early on to include nurses, practice managers, and lay representatives.[56] Accordingly, some of these groups have changed their title to primary care audit groups (PCAG) and widened their brief to support a range of quality initiatives which will now include clinical governance. As in most other activities, staff within community trusts have had completely different audit agendas and support infrastructures. There are examples of collaborative audit[57] but these tend to be in the minority. PCGs need to explore how to develop audit that bridges the divides between organizations just as the care experienced by the older person does. Even more challenging will be to develop audit that crosses the health and social care divide. Perhaps the development of 'care pathways' in primary care settings can offer one way forward.

The experience of the nineties would suggest that health care professionals have different attitudes to audit and can be divided into the following groupings:

- the enthusiasts
- those who consider it routine
- those who are cynical and resist
- and those who opt out.

While negative attitudes[58] and concerns about the burden it places on already busy practitioners[59] have been reported, others argue that participation is widespread.[60] The evidence for the impact of audit alone on changing clinical activities is weak,[61] but there is some evidence that audit combined with educational strategies can produce significant changes in professional behaviours.[62] In general practice it has been noted that there is a relationship between practice size and audit activity – the more partners the more likely there is audit activity,[63] which is presumably a function of greater resources.

The association between more collaborative teamworking in practices and multi-disciplinary audit activities has also been noted.[64]

Below we give some recent texts on how to undertake clinical audit:

- Fraser R, Lakhani M & Baker R *Evidence-based audit in general practice* Butterworth Heinneman, Oxford 1998.
- National Health Service Executive *Achieving effective practice: a clinical effectiveness and research information pack for nurses, midwives and health visitors.* HMSO Clinical Effectiveness Resource Folder, HMSO, London 1998.
- National Centre for Clinical Audit *Clinical audit action pack, version 2* NCCA, London 1997.

The nineties have witnessed the call for evidence-based health care as part of a wider clinical effectiveness initiative which at times has seemed almost evangelical. In 1998 the Clinical Standards Advisory Group reported that the most visible sign of work on clinical effectiveness was the production of guidelines,[65] that is, statements of good practice based on research evidence. However, the challenges remain that strong scientific evidence is not available to support a great deal of current practice, and that much 'caring' as opposed to 'curing' activity is not amenable to testing via experimentation based on scientific trials. We touched on the limitations of the guidelines approach to the primary care of older people in the previous chapter. The Scottish Intercollegiate Guidelines Network proposed a system of acknowledging the strength of the evidence used in guidelines.[66] This described three levels: the strongest evidence based on systematic reviews of randomized control trials, the next level based on evidence from other types of quantitative experiments, and lastly recognized expert opinion. The academics at the Eli Lilly Centre for Audit have echoed this in devising audit protocols which specify 'must do' elements based on strong evidence with important impacts on outcomes, while 'should do' elements have less impact on outcome and less strong evidence.[67] The search for best available evidence to base their activities and audit criteria is becoming easier for busy health care professionals with the publication of systematic reviews and clinical guidance endorsed at a national level. The National Institute of Clinical Excellence has been established to provide a single focus for the production of evidence-based clinical guidance on effective interventions. The list below shows some useful contact points for accessing this guidance and associated audit packages:

- your local primary care audit group
- your local trust audit department or clinical governance committee
- The Nursing and Midwifery Audit Information Service, RCN, 20 Cavendish Square, London W1M OAB. E-mail:dqi@rcn.org.uk
- Eli Lily National Clinical Audit Centre, Dept. of General Practice and Primary Health Care, Leicester University, Leicester General Hospital, Gwendolyn Road, Leicester LE5 4PW. E-mail:clinaudit@le.ac.uk.

At the same time national service frameworks are being heralded as 'care blueprints',[68] setting out what patients can expect to receive from the NHS in major care areas or disease groups.

The conundrum remains however: while on the one hand national guidelines solve the time problem for primary care professionals, on the other hand
professionals are more likely to implement professional practices prescribed in
guidelines if they have a sense of ownership and played a part in determining
them.[69] In fact, the reasons why we professionals do or do not change our professional behaviour is imperfectly understood. In this light, multifaceted
approaches[70,71] alongside guideline or protocol development would seem to
make the most sense, including:

- capitalizing on the influence of local opinion leaders
- providing role models
- innovative models of continuing education
- using computer-aided decision support systems.

In the complex provision of health and social care for older people, there
are many who are beginning to argue that the clinical guidance for effective
practice is not enough and that maps (locally negotiated) are needed to detail
what should happen during the care of a person with a certain condition or set
of conditions, and *when*, but more importantly *by who* and in *what sequence*.
These sorts of maps are care pathways or shared-care protocols, and we provide examples of them in the clinical chapters.

Audit methodologies

Most methods of audit involve the collection of data on the agreed criteria for
a sample of patients. Collection of data from existing (preferably computerized) records significantly reduces the burden of audit but depends on accurate record keeping. It is worth pointing out here that there is potentially yet
another linguistic chasm between medicine and nursing. In nursing, the word
'standard'[72] has been used to describe what the medical audit literature
describes as criteria. 'Standard setting' has been a widespread prolific activity
across nursing services since the eighties.[73] The medical audit literature
describes 'standards' as a target level of performance usually expressed as a
percentage. So the statement 'the diabetic patient will have their feet checked
annually for foot lesions and dermatological abnormalities' would be a standard to some but a criteria to others, who would view the addition of 'in 100%
of cases' as the standard. Teams and audit groups beware the language differences! These types of audit are also applied to monitoring non-clinical activities such as waiting times and response rates in relevant user/patient charters.

Critical incident and significant event analysis

This is a type of audit based on a single important event in the care of an individual from which the professionals try and understand what happened in the
process of the care for that event to happen. The purpose of this is to change
or rectify the elements that led to the event so that it is less likely to happen in
the future. This type of review of performance is based on the premise that the

team can learn and adapt, in a climate of no blame.[74] It is a process that has been adopted in many risk management strategies where it is recognized that it involves the team, the situation, and the organization which needs to enhance its performance.[75] Pringle describes significant event auditing as less intellectually rigorous and less mechanistic than conventional clinical audit. He argues that it has a strong emotional content which makes its link to the change in professional behaviour potentially much more powerful, a view supported elsewhere.[76,77] In this process events deemed significant, which include death, emergencies, and clinical and administrative occurrences are selected for consideration. Meetings of the team are arranged to discuss the selected event through a case presentation and analysis of it, and on the basis of the structured discussion, decisions are made and recorded. This may lead to subsequent conventional audits. A summary of the strengths and weaknesses of this form of audit are reproduced in Box 4.4.

The following are suggestions for the types of significant events in the health care of older people a primary health care team could consider:

- a patient or carer complaint
- a patient suffering a fracture following a fall
- readmission to hospital within two weeks of discharge
- sudden unexpected death
- a cerebrovascular accident
- attempted suicide
- new cancer diagnosis

Box 4.4 *Strengths and weaknesses of significant event analysis*[78]

Potential strengths

- outcomes are focused
- high emotional appeal
- high face validity
- deals with practical and relevant issues
- may require less preparatory effort (than conventional audit)
- less exclusively reliant on written records
- feedback is immediate, from known peers
- builds trust and improves teamworking
- raises interface and team issues

Potential drawbacks

- may be rather superficial
- may be threatening
- emotionally demanding
- may require additional training
- can expose team or interface issues that are difficult to resolve
- requires discipline in group discussions, particularly concluding discussions, with clear points.

- registration of a diabetic person as partially blind
- failure of a service to carry out a home visit as agreed
- neglect or abuse by family member, informal carer, or formal carer
- members of the team upset by an incident or ongoing events.

Views from the patients and users

As our earlier case study demonstrated, the patient perspective is important for a team to understand all elements of its performance, and the differences in perception of performance between the professional and the patient should not be underestimated. There is often significant difference in views between patients and their GPs about the doctors' ability to put patients at ease and to offer explanations and advice on treatment.[79] All the quality policy initiatives of the nineties we have been describing so far have encouraged the inclusion of patient perspectives; for this reason teams need to acknowledge this as a useful source of evaluation of their work and find ways of incorporating it into their planning. The first and simplest step is the addition of a review of patient appreciation and patients' complaints to team or audit meetings. Primary care groups might like to consider how the current separate mechanism for collating these between general practice, trusts, and social services could be brought together. More proactive approaches can be incorporated into audit projects with specific questions recording patient perspectives. Surveys of patient satisfaction have been popular forms of audit according to some medical audit advisory groups' (MAAG) reports.[80] The difficulties of undertaking satisfaction surveys are well documented, particularly with older people who may not wish to appear critical of the services upon which they depend. Advice on these and other methods such as focus groups, observation techniques, and patient diaries can be found in the publications below:

- King's Fund. *Information on obtaining the views of users of primary health care services: consumer feedback resource.* King's Fund Centre, London 1991.
- Baker R, Hearnshaw H, Cooper A *et al. A guide to choosing and using patient questionnaires in general practice.* 1994 Eli Lilly Centre for Clinical Audit, Leicester University 1994.
- College of Health *Ask the patient: new approaches to consumer audit feedback in general practice.* The College of Health, London 1991.
- Kelson M *Consumer involvement in clinical audits and outcomes: a review of developments and issues in the identification of good practice.* College of Health, London 1994.

This chapter has outlined key elements in developing an infrastructure for quality health care. In a sense, the following checklist provides a summary and then poses some key questions for a research agenda.

Basic elements for infrastructure development in the care of older people in the community include:

(1) Identification of the core team of people involved
(2) Written team annual objectives of the service to be offered
(3) Agreed methods of communication processes, including clinical review meetings
(4) Annual plan for monitoring the provision and quality , including information requirements and review meetings
(5) Quarterly plan for networking and education events
(6) Annual social gathering to celebrate the achievements, mourn the death of long-standing patients, and reflect on how to provide an even better service next year.

Questions for a primary care of older people research agenda include:

- What types of multidisciplinary working improve the health and social outcomes for older people and their carers?
- Which team organizational factors have the greatest impact on the outcome for older people?
- What are the most effective methods of incorporating older people's views in the audit and team effectiveness processes?
- Does joint professional/service documentation improve communication?
- What scope is there for patient-held records in improving communication?

A number of issues need to be developed further in the context of the population-based approaches and the clinical governance developments in primary care, which we do in the last section of the book. Having set the scene for development of primary care for older people, we now return to the individual patient care and management, to put theory into practice.

References

1 Royal College of Nursing and Royal College of General Practice *Report of the joint working party on the primary health care team*. RGCP, London 1961.

2 Department of Health and Social Security *The Primary Health Care Team Report of the Joint Working Group of the Standing Medical Advisory Committee and the Standing Nursing and Midwifery Committee* (chairman W Harding). DHSS, London 1981.

3 Abel R *Staff implications of schemes of attachment of local health authority staff (HV and home nursing) to general practitioners*. Study No.1. DHSS Social Science Research Unit, HMSO 1969.

4 DHSS *Neighbourhood nursing – a focus for care*. HMSO, London 1986.

5 Marsh G & Kaim Caudle P *Teamwork in general practice*. Croom-Helm, London 1976.

6 Gregson B, Cartilidge A, Bond J *et al. Interprofessional collaboration in primary health care organisations*. Occasional paper 52. Royal College of General Practitioners, London 1991.

7 Audit Commission *Homeward bound* Audit Commission, London 1992.

8 The NHS and Community Care Act 1990. HMSO, London 1990.

9 Department of Health *The NHS: modern and dependable* (Cm.3852). The Stationery Office, London 1998.

10 Department of Health *Personal medical services pilots of the NHS (Primary Care Act)1997.* EL (97)27.

11 Department of Health. *Partnership in action: a discussion document.* HMSO, London 1998.

12 Editorial The latest official statistics. *Employing Nurses* 1996; **September:** 10–11.

13 Green S A pivot for the practice. *Nursing Times* 1993; **89**:(46):42–4.

14 Knott M Integrated nursing teams: developments in general practice. *Community Practitioner* 1999; **72**(2):23–4.

15 Koperski M, Rogers S, Drennan V. Nurse practitioners in general practice: an inevitable progression? *British Journal of General Practice* 1997; **November**:696–7.

16 Pearson P & Jones K *Primary care–opportunities and threats. British Medical Journal* 1997; **314**(7083): 817–20.

17 Firth-Cozens J Celebrating teamwork. *Quality in Health Care 1998;* **7**:S3–S7.

18 Gilmore M , Bruce N, & Hunt M The work of the nursing team in general practice. Council for the Education and Training of Health visitors, London 1974.

19 Royal College of General Practitioners *The nature of general medical practice.* Report from General Practice: No. 27. RCGP, London 1996.

20 Gilmore M, Bruce N, & Hunt M, op. cit.

21 Dawson S *Analysing Organisations.* Macmillan Press, London 1992.

22 Adelaide Medical Centre Primary Health Care Team A primary health care team manifesto. *British Journal of General Practice* 1991; **41**:(342):31–3.

23 Pritchard P & Pritchard J *Teamwork for primary and shared care: a practical work book* (2nd edn). Oxford University Press, Oxford 1994.

24 Carnell C A *Managing change in organisations.* Prentice Hall, London 1990.

25 Poulton B & West M. A Failure of Function. *Teamwork in primary health care. J. Inter professional Care* 1997; **11**(2): 205–16.

26 Ovretveit J *Essentials of multidisciplinary organisation.* Brunel University, Uxbridge 1988.

27 Gregson B, Cartilidge A, & Bond J (1991), op. cit.

28 Hudson B Joint working: local differences. *Health Service Journal* 1997; **137**:31–3.

29 See for example Gregson *et al.,* 1991, op. cit.

30 Pritchard P In Owens P, Carrier J, & Horder J (eds) *Inter-professional issues in community and primary health care.* Macmillan Press, London 1995.

31 Pritchard P (1995), op.cit.

32 Firth-Cozens J (1998), op. cit..

33 Huntington J *Social work and general medical practice: collaboration or conflict.* George Alan & Unwin, London 1981.

34 Zairi M & Mathew A *TQM in primary care: an evaluation.* European Centre for Total Quality Management, University of Bradford 1993.

35 Lambert D Developing primary health care teams. *Primary Health Care Management 1991;* **12**:2–3.

36 Lawrence M & Packwood T Adapting total quality management for general practice: evaluation of a programme. Quality in Health Care 1996; **5**:151–8.

37 Gillam S & Miller R *COPC – a public health experiment in primary care.* Kings Fund, London 1997.

38 Lewis R & Williams S *LIZ: a legacy for London. Health Service Journal* 1998; **108**:24–6.

39 Bryar R & Bytheway B *Changing primary health care. The Team Care Valley's experience.* Blackwell Science Limited, Oxford 1996.

40 Pearson P & Jones K Primary care–opportunities and threats. *British Medical Journal* 1997; **314**(7083):817–20.

41 Dorset FHSA. Primary care team development: final report 1992.

42 Burns F *Information for health: an information strategy for the modern NHS 1998 –2005.* HMSO, London 1998.

43 Millburn A *Patient records.* House of Commons Official Report (Hansard) 1998, Feb 9; Col 59.

44 Audit Commission *Comparing notes: a study of information management in community trusts.* Audit Commission, London 1997.

45 Burns F NHS information strategy, op. cit., p. 73.

46 Redfern S & Norman I *The validity of quality assessment iInstruments in nursing: final report to the department of health.* Section 1.2, p.3. Nursing Research Unit, King's College, London 1994.

47 Donabedian A Evaluating the quality of medical care. *Millbank Memorial Fund Quarterly* 1996; **44**:166–206.

48 Maxwell R Quality assessment in health. *British Medical Journal 1984;* **288**:1470–2.

49 Maxwell R Dimensions of quality revisited: from thought to action. Quality in Health Care 1992; **1**:171–7.

50 NHSE *A first-class service: quality in the new NHS.* HMSO, London 1998.

51 Cm.4169 White Paper *Modernising social services.* Section 7. The Stationery Office, London 1998.

52 Health Service Circular 1988/228:LAC (98) 32 *The NHS Modern and Dependable Primary Care Groups Delivering the Agenda.*

53 HSC 1999/065 Clinical Governance: Quality in the new NHS. 1999.

54 Health Service Circular 1988/228:LAC (98) 32 *The NHS: modern and dependable primary care groups delivering the agenda.*

55 Baker R, Hearnshaw H, Cooper A Assessing the work of medical audit advisory groups in promoting audit in general practice. *Quality in Health Care* 1995; 4:234–9.

56 Humphrey C & Berrow D Developing the role of the medical audit advisory groups. *Quality in health Care* 1993; 2:232–8.

57 Berrow D & Humphrey C Working together for quality improvement. *Audit Trends* 1996; 4(2) 53–58.

58 Chambers R Bowyers S & Campbell I Investigation into the attitudes of general practitioners in Staffordshire to medical audit. *Quality in Health Care* 1996; 5(1):13–19.

59 Black N & Thompson E Obstacles to medical audit: British doctors speak. *Social Science and Medicine 1993;* 36:849–56.

60 Lewis C & Coombes D Is general practice audit alive and well? The view from Portsmouth. *British Journal of General Practice* 1996; 46:735–6.

61 Thomson R & Barton A Is audit running out of steam? *Quality in Health Care* 1994; 3:225–9.

62 Fraser R, Lakhani M, & Baker R *Evidence-based audit in general practice.* Butterworth Heinneman, Oxford 1998.

63 Baker R, Robertson N, Farooqi A Audit in general practice: factors influencing participation. *British Medical Journal* 1995; 311:31–4.

64 Davies C *et al.* Factors influencing audit in general practice. *International Journal of Health Care Quality Assurance* 1996; 9(5):5–9.

65 Clinical Standards Advisory Group *Summary of the Report on Clinical Effectiveness* (using stroke as an example). Department of Health, London 1998.

66 Scottish Intercollegiate Guidelines Network *Developing national guidelines.* SIGN pamphlet, 1995.

67 Fraser R, Lakhani M & Baker R, op. cit., p. 8.

68 National Health Service Executive *A first-class service – quality in the new NHS.* Summary. HMSO, London 1998.

69 Grimshaw JM, Freemantle N, Wallace S, *et al.* Developing and implementing clinical practice guidelines. *Quality in Health Care* 1995; 4:55–64.

70 Haines A, & Jones R Implementing findings of research. *British Medical Journal* 1994; 308:1488–92.

71 Kitson A, Ahmed LB, Harvey G From research to practice: one organisational model for promoting research-based practice. *Journal of Advanced Nursing* 1996; 23:430–40.

72 Redfern S & Norman I The validity of quality assessment instruments in nursing; final report to the Department of Health. Section 1.2, p.3. Nursing Research Unit, King's College London 1994.

73 Redfern S & Norman I, op. cit.

74 Pringle M Bradley C, Carmichael CM *Significant event analysis.* Occasional paper 70. Royal College of General Practitioners, London 1995.

75 Reason J Understanding adverse events: the human factors. *Quality in Health Care* 1995; **4**:(2):80–8.

76 Benett IJ & Danczak AF Terminal care: improving teamwork in primary care using significant event analysis. *European Journal of Cancer Care 1994;* **3**(2):54–7.

77 Redpath L Stacey A, Pugh E Use of critical incident technique in primary care in the audit of deaths by suicide. *Quality in Health Care* 1997; **6**:25–8.

78 Pringle M Bradley C, Carmichael CM (1995), op. cit.

79 Rashid A Forman W, Jagger C, & Mann R Consultations in general practice: a comparison of patients' and doctors' satisfaction. *British Medical Journal* 1989; **299**:1015–6.

80 Baker R & Streatfield J What type of general practice do patients prefer? Exploration of practice characteristics influencing patient satisfaction. *British Journal of General Practice* 1995; **455**:654–9.

CHAPTER FIVE

Disability, functional loss, and falls

Mr and Mrs H were woken up not long after midnight by the Remote Monitoring Centre linked to Mrs H.'s 82-years-old mother's alarm systems. Mrs H.'s mother, Ivy, had fallen over in her bathroom an hour or so before, and had only just reached the alarm pull to get help, having left her alarm pendant beside her bed. She had taken her sleeping tablets at 8 o'clock but then decided not to go to bed, but to watch television instead. When she finally got up to use the lavatory before sleeping, she had lost her balance turning in the bathroom. It was her third fall in the same number of months.

When admitted to a general medical ward in the local hospital just after dawn on the same day, Mrs H.'s mother was examined, had X-rays of her chest and (painful) right hip, received oxygen, and had an intravenous line inserted. She understated her cigarette consumption at 10–15 daily, not the 30 that her family knew she smoked, and said that she only had a nip of Bailey's at night to help her sleep, although her consumption was a bottle a week. Her BMI was recorded as 31, but no further action was taken about this. Her oedema up to her knees was noted, as were her use of frusemide, digoxin, and temazepam. Her X-rays showed no bone injury, her mood became exuberant in the busy atmosphere of the ward, her haemotology and biochemistry results came back as normal, and she was discharged home to the very attentive care of her family and neighbours, with support planned by community nurses and social services.

This happened in January 1999. The increasingly angry and frustrated family returned to their tasks of caring for an increasingly demanding and dependent relative, relieved by the support they were getting from health and social services, but saddened that they could not get Ivy's general practitioner to visit her at home. A friend suggested that they remove all bottles of alcohol and dissuade friends and neighbours from buying replacements, and that the temazepam could be confiscated, which they did.

In primary care we are good at dealing with some kinds of disability (or functional loss) but not with others. Complex situations, like Ivy's, test our ability to understand and respond to patients' needs in ways that rapidly reveal our limited knowledge, the poor coordination of different services and disciplines, and the priorities we give to different sorts of patients and their problems. Ivy's rapid return to some kind of normality was a relief to the hard-pressed ward staff, who could discharge her and free her bed for someone less jovial and less well supported. No one took away her benzodiazepine medication, let alone stopped prescribing it, and her normal blood tests and fracture-free films allowed her pathologies – which had made her fall three times in three months – to be removed from the clinical agenda. The integrating of acute care and rehabilitation in single, multi-purpose wards during the eighties has shifted the balance of activity away from rehabilitation, especially given the continued pressure for high throughput of patients.[1] Community services, responsive after an injection of funds designed to avert a winter bed crisis, worked wonders in supporting her in her home, but given their historic legacy of under-resourcing, were as unable as the hospital ward to initiate rehabilitation.[2]

Falling is a common experience for older people, but for most in the community it usually has only short-term consequences, the scenarios like that above being the exception not the rule. About 30% of those aged 65 and over fall each year,[3] the rate rising up to 50% for those aged 80 or more. Most of those living independently who fall never seek medical attention, so the consultation rate with GPs for falls in the 66–80 age group is nine per 1000 people per year, rising to 25 per 1000 amongst those over 80 years of age, a pattern we encountered in Chapter 2. Nevertheless, among people aged 65 and over in England and Wales in 1991, 85% of deaths due to accidents in the home were accounted for by falls.[4] In Scotland alone, in 1991, falls among those 75 years and older accounted for 200 deaths, 5000 hospital admissions, and 13,500 new out-patient visits.[5] Rates of falling increase with rising rates of illness, and are higher in people in residential care, peaking in long-term nursing institutions and geriatric wards. These are also the group at greatest risk of significant injury from falls,[6] with fractured neck of femur a common outcome.

Nevertheless, falls should be viewed as signs and warnings, however minor each fall may be and regardless of the degree of injury, because of the psychological impact of falling, including the fear of future falling,[7] and the risk of further functional deterioration. Falls may be symptoms of underlying disease processes, impairments, and disabilities, but they may also be the causes of disability. If we can understand how falls happen in older people, we can understand the processes of disablement and see how intervention in primary care might alter the risks and consequences of falling. First we need to consider the aetiology of falls, then we can put aetiological information into a dynamic model of disablement. Figure 5.1 below shows how falls fit into a pathological system that readily converts into a vicious spiral of disability.

Postural control is maintained by the integration of proprioceptive, vestibular, and visual signals, at reflex level within the central nervous system, to produce an effective motor response. Damage to any part of this system can cause postural disturbance, yet the system is relatively robust and flexible, so the impact of damage (or ageing) on postural control in any individual is unpredictable. The physiological changes (impairments) which seem important are:

- increases in postural sway with ageing
- increased proprioceptive thresholds

- diminishing accuracy in reproducing and matching joint angles
- declining visual acuity
- diminishing visual contrast sensitivity
- decreasing muscle power
- increased reaction times and muscle activation time
- slower central integration of sensory inputs.

Central integration of sensory input is diminished by anxiety and distraction, which explains why those with a fear of falling have objectively poorer postural control[8] than their less fearful peers, and why falls may be precipitated by changes in routine or in the environment. Small, slow movements require more central integration than faster, larger movements, and are more stressful for posture control systems, as Ivy found when she tried to turn after walking into the bathroom. Illness, not ageing, is the most important factor in disturbing balance, for frail older people have profound changes in balance control compared with healthy older people of the same age. We can conceptualize some of the interrelated factors determining falls, and their consequences, as shown in Figure 5.1.

Case management approaches

The ways in which different problems interact to produce further disability is a disconcerting one, at first glance, and a long way from the comforting linear cascades of biomedicine, but this model offers multiple opportunities for

Figure 5.1 Factors promoting falls.[9]

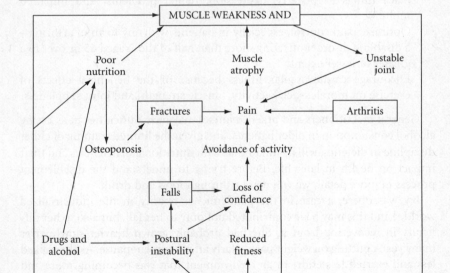

intervention by primary care workers. For example, from Figure 5.1 we can produce the following action plans to fit into a case management approach:

- Check all medication prescribed for older patients, to reduce use of benzodiazepine hypnotics and tranquillizers. We discussed medication review in Chapter 3, and will return to the use of hypnotics and analgesics in relation to disability in the chapter on depression. Here we need only say that use of benzodiazepines can reduce functional ability to the same extent as arthritis, hip fracture, and cardiovascular or chronic lung disease.10

- Ask about alcohol consumption, routinely. Whilst alcohol consumption in the population declines with advancing age,[11] alcohol can play a significant role in the aetiology of falls in some older individuals.

- Make the prevention of osteoporosis a target in primary care. We have discussed the potential for screening for osteoporosis in Chapter 3, but whatever view is taken at practice level about this, there is no reason not to inform patients about the value of taking calcium and vitamin D, of the apparent advantages of long-term hormone replacement therapy for post-menopausal women, and of the protective effects of regular physical activity (brisk walking) on bone. Vitamin D and calcium supplementation in doses up to one-third higher than the recommended daily intake reduced hip fractures by 20% over a three-year period in very old female nursing home residents, either by increasing bone density or by improving muscle function, or both.[12] We will return to promotion of physical activity in Chapters 11 and 12.

- Think about nutrition, which is relatively neglected in primary care despite the fact that undernutrition is a consequence of such commonplace things as poverty, depression, dental problems, and impaired mobility.

- Optimize pain control, especially in patients with any form of arthritis – a disabling disorder affecting more than half of those aged 65 or over to a greater or lesser extent.

- Encourage cardiovascular fitness because of the beneficial effects of exercise on morale, social activity, muscle strength, and joint suppleness.

General practitioners and practice nurses may have difficulties in assessing alcohol consumption in older patients, and given the limited training of either discipline in dietetics, will be unfamiliar with nutritional deficiencies and their impact on health in later life. Before trying to understand the disablement process in more detail, we will detour through food and drink.

Ivy was obese, a case in the pandemic of obesity in the industrialized world,[13] and this may have contributed not only to her fall, but also to her difficulty in recovering from it. She had probably grown heavier slowly, over many years, putting on weight particularly after her menopause. As she walked less and exerted less effort in an environment that was becoming more and more labour-saving, she became unfit and oxidized fat less, so that her unchanging high-fat diet helped her enlarge and further limited her activity.

Fat loss and maintainance of lower fat stores become more difficult with ageing,[13] so her BMI continued to rise even though she tried several short, sharp diets to reduce her weight. Could any of this have been prevented, and is there any intervention now that could reduce Ivy's weight to a level that poses less of a threat to her? The questions are not academic, nor are they specific to this complex patient, for the population is getting heavier and the prevalence of obesity is increasing rapidly, so an increasing number of older people are likely to find themselves in Ivy's position.

The answers lie in understanding that:

- low-energy diets (less food) are no better than low-fat diets in reducing weight in the long term, but are harder to maintain
- physiological adjustment to weight loss produces plateaus in weight loss, especially if the energy disequilibrium is extreme because of sudden dietary change or vigorous exercise
- vigorous exercise – even if possible – produces less fat loss than sustained moderate exercise (such as walking) in unfit people
- sustained small increases in physical activity and reductions in fat content of diets have the greatest impacts.

Had Ivy been encouraged to think in these terms, with a knowledge of what a lower-fat diet is like, and with enough money to buy the right food, she might have avoided the obesity that threatens to trap her in disability.

The opposite problem of undernutrition exists in the older population, but is relatively uncommon in the community, occurring most frequently in the frail, in those needing hospital admission, and in those living in nursing and residential homes. Protein–calorie undernutrition is uncommon amongst healthy older people living autonomously,[14] does not increase with advancing age, with no features of nutrient malabsorption appearing during ageing, in the absence of disease processes.[15] The story amongst frail older people is entirely different. Age-related loss of senses of taste and smell that reduce appetite, dental problems causing difficulties with chewing, impaired ability to purchase and prepare food, and lower overall intake secondary to diminished physical activity all contribute to changing eating habits. Phases of undernutrition and weight loss triggered by life events or illness can accumulate to produce progressive undernutrition, which may not be diagnosed.[16] The population of frail older people therefore experiences a high prevalence of low or marginal nutrition,[17] and between a third and a half of older people admitted to hospital as an emergency have features of undernutrition.[18] The undernourished status of this in-patient population also increases its risks of developing new morbidity when in hospital, even though nutrient intake increases.[19] The contribution of progressive undernutrition to the process of disablement then becomes clear, as the trajectory of a hypothetical patient shown in figure 5.2 demonstrates.

This pattern can be observed if older patients are weighed whenever seen in the surgery or clinic, and their weight charted – current electronic medical records should have a graphing facility that makes trends easy to spot. A

Figure 5.2 The descent into undernutrition.

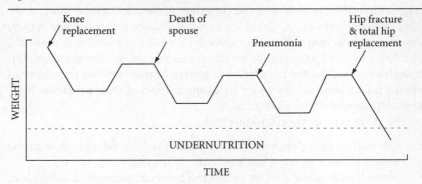

dietary history can be important when progressive weight loss is occurring, and when frailty and disability supervene, but there is no single best method for obtaining this information. One approach is to ask the individual to complete a self-rating scale of the kind shown in Box 5.1.[20]

Box 5.1 *Dietary history – self completion questionnarie*

FOR EACH YES ANSWER, SCORE THE NUMBER IN THE BOX   YES

I have an illness or condition that made me change the kind or amount of food I eat.	2
I eat fewer than two meals a day.	3
I eat few fruits or vegetables, or milk products.	2
I have three or more drinks of beer, spirits, or wine almost everyday.	2
I have tooth or mouth problems that make it hard for me to eat.	2
I do not always have enough money to buy the food I need.	4
I eat alone most of the time.	1
I take three or more prescribed or over-the-counter medicines a day	1
I have lost or gained 10 pounds in weight in the last six months, without wanting to.	2
I am not always physically able to shop, cook, and/or feed myself.	2
TOTAL	

A score of 0–2 suggests no risk of undernutrition, 3–5 a moderate risk, and 6 or more high nutritional risk. This scale has a low specificity, so individuals with high scores require a further review by a practitioner with some awareness of nutrition issues. This may have unexpected beneficial effects.

Mrs G., first encountered in Chapter 2, had concealed her alcohol consumption from the practice nurse doing the 75-and-over check, but completion of the nutrition check-list in the safety of her own home prompted a more honest response. Mrs G. ate most of her meals alone, and had poor teeth because of a lifetime's dental neglect, so she scored 3 and attracted a review by her doctor that demonstrated that she was not suffering with hypoproteinaemia, but was significantly depressed .

Of course, some patients will not find such a self-completion questionnaire easy or possible, so direct assessment by a nurse or doctor using the same questions will be needed. A comprehensive dietary history is likely to be too difficult and time-consuming to be practical in most primary care settings, and belongs to the specialist dietician who should be engaged only when the practitioner has suspicions about undernutrition.

Decreased serum albumin indicates decreased protein intake and reduced protein status, and low levels of albumin are associated with increased morbidity in older people,[21] so simple biochemical testing (along with a full blood count and calcium estimation) are justified as part of routine assessment whenever undernutrition is suspected. A flow chart for assessment of nutritional risk in frail and disabled older patients would then look like that in Figure 5.3.

The role of the dietician is important here for those in primary care groups now considering how to allocate resources to this speciality. In the past, dieticians working in primary care settings have suffered the fate of social workers who worked alongside general practitioners in the eighties (see Chapter 2), with dilution of their specialist input and a tendency to concentrate on the younger rather than older patients. Perhaps highly focused attention to the nutritional status of older people might be a more appropriate deployment of their expertise?

Understanding rehabilitation

Given the complex causes and consequences of falls, where should primary care workers start with any given patient? With Ivy, it is easy to intervene, party because circumstances demand action and partly because some interventions are obvious. What about patients whose problems are not so extreme, like the otherwise fit, 77-year-old man who falls over one day whilst out on a particularly strenuous shopping expedition, or the robust octogenarian woman who has a 'dizzy turn' and falls whilst playing bowls? To understand the significance of their falls we need to understand the trajectory of disability in later life.

Disability is the gap between capability and demand. For Ivy, her need to stay standing was undermined by her ability, when a brain probably impaired by atherosclerosis was also influenced by drugs and alcohol. She demonstrated a disabling process that is summed up in Figure 5.4.[22]

The more factors operating within this model (Figure 5.4), the faster the person is driven towards disability. An older person with no risk factors has only an 8% annual chance of falling, whilst four factors give a 78% risk.[23] This model of the disablement process also allows for some of the paradoxes that we experience in practice. Not all people with impairments are disabled, and

Figure 5.3 *Flowchart for assessment of nutritional risk in frail and disabled older patients.*

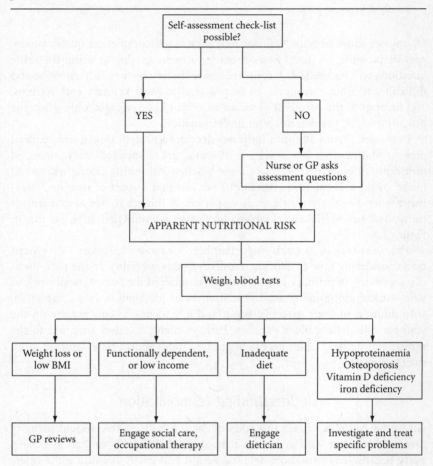

not all disabled people have impairments that are commensurate with their degree of disability. Similarly, medical care – especially medication and surgery – can make disabilities worse as well as better, and efforts at support can reduce independence and ability in some people. It also allows us to plan interventions at different levels, taking into account the environmental circumstances and personal characteristics of each individual.

There are, then, four basic steps to disability assessment in primary care:[24]

(1) characterize the disabilities
(2) identify the causal impairments
(3) determine the disease processes underlying impairments
(4) identify other contributing factors, in demand and capability.

This is a framework for case management, for it creates a hierarchy of topics to work through in order to solve the individual patient's problems. For example, characterizing the disability requires determination of:

Figure 5.4 The disablement process.

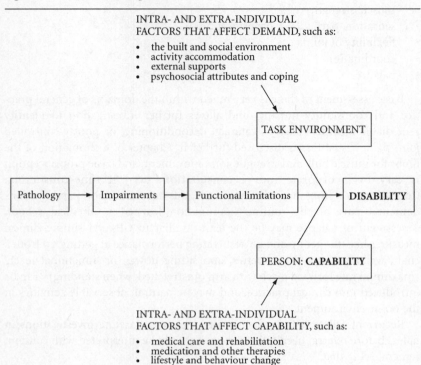

- its severity, in terms of limitations in activity, need for assistance
- the time-scale of its evolution
- associated clinical symptoms and signs, including those of affective disorders and cognitive impairment (see Chapter 9)
- compensations and adaptations, such as equipment or avoidance of tasks
- other disabilities – the patient unable to walk to the corner shop may not be able to get in or out of their bath either.

In the case of Ivy, the disability – in the sense of not being able to stay standing – was severe, requiring hospital admission, and apparently had a short-time scale of three months. However, the associated signs, like forgetting about taking hypnotics at the right time or wearing the alarm pendant, suggest a longer course and possibly underlying cognitive impairment. She already had aids to daily living organized around her risk of falling, and almost certainly was unable to carry out more difficult tasks such as shopping and home care.

Identifying the underlying causes of disability appears daunting, for there are at least 50 different diseases that can affect walking, but it becomes easier if causation is sought at the level of impairment first. There are six basic impairments that can impact on walking and contribute to falls:

- vision, as described above
- muscle strength
- sensation, particularly proprioception
- flexibility of joints
- coordination
- balance.

Basic assessment of these is very much within the domains of general practice and community nursing, and allows further investigation to identify remediable disorders such as cataract, deconditioning, or poorly controlled joint pain. Visual loss is discussed further in Chapter 6. Examination of the limbs for muscle bulk and strength, joint movement, and basic proprioception is easy to incorporate into a consultation, even if time-consuming. Coordination testing may take more time, but not much more, and is a fundamental part of the routine examination learned in medical school. Assessment of balance may be the least familiar to GPs, yet simple clinical measures like the 'get up and go' test (rating performance at getting up from a chair, walking about three metres, and sitting down) or 'functional reach' (maximum safe forward reach with arm outstretched, when standing)[25] can be introduced into clinical practice, and may be natural, observable activities in the home environment.

Recurrent falls call for specialist investigation. Baseline investigations in fallers before referral need to be done but should be interpreted with caution, remembering that:

- postural dizziness is not usually associated with postural hypotension, but is associated with falls, probably through a shared central impairment secondary to cerebral atherosclerosis
- postural hypotension is a less powerful predictor of falls than dizziness
- arrhythmias occur in 15% of asymptomatic older people, and are no more common in fallers than in non-fallers.

Demand and capability factors can be assessed with the mnemonic SAFE:

- Social support and, Safety in the home
- Attitude (motivation, expectations, culture) and Affective disorders
- Finances
- Environment and Education.

Interventions to reduce impairments may be specific to the underlying diseases, highly focused, and aimed at correcting functional loss, or part of multifactorial interventions designed to alter a number of factors contributing to functional loss and disability. We discuss primary and secondary prevention of cardiovascular diseases in Chapter 7, pulmonary rehabilitation in Chapter 10, and assessment and treatment of visual and hearing loss in Chapter 6. Here we will review focused and multifactorial interventions against falls.

Multifactorial interventions

Promoting physical exercise is in itself not sufficient to reduce the incidence of falls in unselected community-dwelling older people,[26] and even when designed to prevent osteoporosis may have the unintended and undesirable effect of increasing the falls rate.[27] On the other hand, supervised exercise programmes aimed at women aged 80 or more, or older people with measurable but mild deficits in strength and balance, are followed by lower rates of falling.[28] Semi-independent residents of nursing homes (probably similar in functional impairment to Ivy) showed no reduction in fall rates, at least in the short term, after balance, flexibility, and resistance training.[29]

Combining exercise training with medication review, assessment of environmental hazards, and other relevant interventions does appear to reduce the rate of falling, at least in those at high risk or who have fallen already.[28] This is one of the few examples of an effective multifactorial intervention, although as we shall see it is a form of tertiary or even quaternary prevention — we are a long way from knowing if primary prevention of falls, or of any disability other than those consequent on stroke, is feasible. Home assessment of disability and education in risk areas carried out by community nurses or trained volunteers, with referral to the general practitioner when appropriate, reduces the fall rate compared with assessment and education alone.[28] Similarly, identification of accident and emergency (A&E) attenders who have fallen, with referral and follow-up, reduces fall rates. Finally, multifactorial assessment and intervention for residents of nursing homes who have fallen previously reduces the subsequent fall rate, whilst hip protectors attached to clothing appear to prevent femoral neck fractures.

If we look at Ivy's case again we can see what could and should be done to minimize her future risks of falling and sustaining injury, and of further disablement. Imagine that you are her new GP, practice or community nurse, hearing her story and picking up her problems for the first time. The checklist that you could draw up might look like that in table 5.1.

There is a lot to learn about Ivy before an appropriate package of interventions and support can be put in place with, and for, her and her family. Whilst some of these interventions have become obvious from constructing the grid in the light of the evidence about avoiding falls, we still need to know where she is on the trajectory of disability. Does she have moderate dementia, amplified by alcohol and hypnotic medication, with the likelihood of progressive decline and increasing need for continuous care, probably in a residential setting? Or does she have cognitive impairment induced by alcohol and benzodiazepines, muscle weakness due to deconditioning, and a fatalistic approach to her slow deterioration? The two possibilities will generate different management plans, and require different kinds of input from different professionals and agencies.

Fatalistic attitudes towards disability are common in public and professionals alike, and the common perception of disability is one of unrelenting and unstoppable decline. This is not true for the common disabilities, as we

Table 5.1

Assessment	Finding	Intervention
Severity of disability	Severe, needing hospital admission on one occasion	High risk, so multifactorial assessment appropriate
Time-scale of functional decline	Apparently short, but underlying changes probably have a longer history	A more detailed informant history about functional loss might clarify
Associated symptoms & signs	Heart failure and cognitive impairment are possibilities and medication needs reviewing	Investigate both, withdraw benzodiazepine
Compensations & adaptions	Alarm system organized already, and support from family appears extensive	What can Ivy actually do as opposed to what she does do?
Related disabilities	Problems with hygiene and locomotor Incontinence a possibility	Assess (see Chapter 8)
Vision	Not known	Assess (see Chapter 6)
Strength	Unable to get up after fall, so upper and lower limb strength reduced	Supervised and tailored exercise programme likely to be beneficial
Sensation	Unknown	Assess with specialis input from geriatrician, physiotherapist, or occupational therapist
Flexibility	Unknown	
Coordination	Unknown	
Balance	Compromised	Occupational therapist
Social support	Intensive and extensive family and neighbours, plus social services	Is this inadvertently masking remediable medical causes of impairment, and contributing to dependance?

Table 5.1 *Continued*

Assessment	Finding	Intervention
Safe Home	Unknown	Check (see below)
Attitude	Unknown	Informant history needed.
Affective disorder?	Unknown	Depression assessment needed (see Chapter 9)
Finances	Unknown	Social assessment has been done, so this should have been covered
Enviroment	Unknown	Review with social services
Education	Unknown	How much does she know about her need for medication; her disability?

shall see later in this chapter, but it is also untrue of complex and seemingly overwhelming problems like those facing Ivy and her family.

Although the prevalence of disability increases rapidly after the age of 80 years, and frail older women live longer than frail older men, between 10% and 25% of the over-80 age group can show improvements in functional ability over a six-year period.[30] The fluctuating weight of the hypothetical patient shown earlier in this chapter is analogous to the fluctuations that occur in functional ability in most individuals with disability, contradicting the perception that disability is inexorably progressive and that the glidepath at the end of life is a smooth, sometimes steep, downward curve.

If the trajectory of disability is important to planning care, how can we conceptualize it for every disabled patient? The original model works well if we introduce feedback loops that allow existing disabilities to create new diseases, impairments and functional losses, and launch new disablement processes (Figure 5.5).

Ivy may have restricted her recreational walking over a long period of time because of painful arthritis, for which she did not seek further medical help after being told that she had to 'live with it' (the disability). This relative inactivity slowly reduced her cardiopulmonary function (with feedback effects on impairment), further reducing her mobility and her social activities (functional

Figure 5.5 Feedback loops in the disablement process.

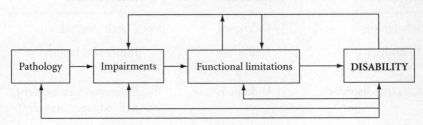

Secondary conditions and dysfunctions in a disablement process

Launch of new disablement processes

limitations and disability). This is an example of secondary dysfunction arising within an existing disablement process. However, demoralized by persistent pain, by her dwindling ability to get around, and by a narrower life than she wanted, she increased her alcohol intake and pressured her doctor into prescribing hypnotics for the sleep disturbance induced by pain, distress, and excess alcohol. The subsequent cognitive impairment added to her functional limitations and produced a new disability – falling. As the feedback loops operate to further promote her existing disability, and perhaps generate new ones, Ivy will move towards a state of unstable disability, or frailty.

Frailty

Frailty is best regarded as a condition or syndrome which results from a multi-system reduction in reserve capacity, to the extent that a number of physiological systems are close to, or past, the threshold of symptomatic clinical failure. The frail person is at increased risk of disability or death from minor external stresses.[31] The ability of the frail older individual depends on the maintenance of key capacities required for successful interaction with the environment, and these are predictable given our model of the disablement process:

- musculoskeletal function
- aerobic capacity
- cognitive and integrative neurological function
- nutritional state.

A comprehensive assessment that views the individual within this framework is likely to draw attention to neglected clinical domains such as nutrition, lower limb strength, and balance, and favour non-pharmacological interventions such as dietary supplements, social activity, and exercise programmes.

How will primary care services cope with the assessment and management of disability and its risks, given the complexities of impairment, functional loss, and the disablement process? Disability rises with age, and the population of the very old is increasing. Primary care services are already stretched meeting demand and developing anticipatory care for a limited range of chronic conditions, primarily in younger age groups. Specialist medical services may not be able to cope with the complexities of disability, and fail as they did with Ivy. Hers was not an isolated case but probably typical of busy acute general medical and even geriatric wards, where performing comprehensive assessments of multifactorial conditions may not be practical, and cannot easily be made so even with the introduction of check-lists that act as decision supports for recognition of disability.[32] If the specialist services are unable to solve this problem, how can we? Perhaps the negative response to the 75-and-over screening programme described in Chapter 2 had even more justification than we described, for no service should attempt to meet need without adequate intellectual or material resources.

This gloom is misplaced. Ivy has many problems, as do her family, and they deserve better than they get, but she is not typical of her peers, nor of older people with disabilities. Epidemiology corrects the perspective biased by experience and anecdote, and the epidemiology of disability in later life is not threatening. Two important themes stand out:

(1) Trends in disability-free life expectancy as a proportion of life expectancy in old age do not show that increased survival is being bought at the expense of a pandemic of dementia and disability.[33]
(2) Impairment explains only a small amount of the disability in the older population, and most impairments act individually, with few operating in combination.[34]

We are better equipped to deal with disability than we think. The greater the disability – the restrictions on an individual in engaging in normal activities – the greater the reduction in control over life experienced by that individual and their stress and depression.[35] Adapting to the reduced physical capacity of ageing – and the sometimes dramatically reduced capacity of disablement – involves invoking cognitive strategies to maintain a sense of control over important life outcomes.[36] These strategies will depend on the individuals own perceptions of health and illness, which we discussed in Chapter 1, but also on the nature of their illness or disability. For example, individual's disabled by one or other form of cancer may tend towards a coping strategy in which they:

- compare themselves with less fortunate others
- selectively focus on attributes that make them appear advantaged
- create hypothetically worse worlds
- construe benefits from the victimizing event or disease
- manufacture normative standards of adjustment that make their own adjustment appear normal.[37]

Other disabilities may produce different patterns, with affected individuals seeing themselves better off than non-disabled peers, partly by selectively focusing on attributes that give them advantages (brain not brawn) or where they can excel – in the quality of their relationships, awareness of others needs, and so on.[38] Who has not heard an older patient with multiple problems say 'I have to be grateful, there are many worse off than me' ?

Interventions that limit the impact of disability may be as much based on psychology as on medical or surgical treatments, but we are better acquainted with the latter. For example, knee replacement is now a reliable therapeutic option for those disabled by arthritis, but is not widely available to those aged 75 and over, and should certainly figure in the commissioning plans of primary care groups.[39] We also know that work with disabled older people depends on:

- understanding the patient's and carer's perceptions of the cause and probable course of their disability
- aiming interventions at both patients and care-givers because of the spillover effects of positive and negative beliefs, behaviours, and moods
- an appreciation of the unique temporal course of different illnesses and disabilities
- identification of those at highest risk of negative outcomes – women care-givers, those with small social networks, those with histories of depression or conflictual relationships
- identification about present or anticipated financial problems.[38]

Whilst the recognition of disability attributable to worsening osteoarthritis of the knee may lead to pressure for more resources in orthopaedic surgery to perform the procedures now seen as effective, how many primary care practitioners would think about diverting resources into cognitive behavioural therapy, family therapy, or benefits advice? Logically we should because the epidemiology of disability is simpler than we think.

A population perspective

Ivy is an uncommon patient, and her likes will not increase in number to such an extent that services will not be able cope – unless services are already inadequate to meet current levels of need. Here a community study by Kempen and colleagues[34] is important for primary care practitioners, for the light it throws on the disablement process as it affects an ageing population as a whole. The complex model of the disablement process applies to complex situations, which are not common (although they increase in prevalence with advancing age[40]), and must be simplified for the usual pattern of disability in the community. Figure 5.6 (derived from Kempen's work) is a suggestion of how disability develops for most older adults who experience it, with solid lines representing main effects and dotted lines the weaker influences.

Most of the time mobility and depression are the keys to understanding disability, with impairment of vision and hearing playing relatively minor roles in the disablement process. Now we know why the link between impairment and disability can be weak, because depression impairs performance, and we also know where to concentrate clinical effort – on maintaining and improving mobility first, on understanding and responding to depression second, and

Figure 5.6 *Disability in whole populations: critical causal factors.*

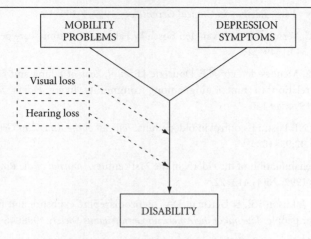

on assessing vision and hearing third. We will pursue these themes in the following chapters, but not before suggesting an agenda about disability for PCGs to consider (Box 5.2).

BOX 5.2 *Addressing disability – five questions for primary care groups*

1.   How will the PCG rehabilitate rehabilitation? Through contracts changes with hospitals to re-emphasize rehabilitation, and even the return of rehabilitation wards? Through use of community hospitals as rehabilitation centres? Through diversion of resources to community-based rehabilitation teams?

2.   What training needs are there in primary care that will equip practitioners for assessment of nutrition, hearing, and vision?

3.   Who will promote physical activity amongst older people, how, and where?

4.   What case management mechanisms need to be put in place at practice level for optimal management of uncommon, complex problems such as posed by Ivy.

5.   What changes are needed in electronic medical records to capture the data needed to profile disability in individuals and in whole populations?

References

1 Young J, Robinson J, & Dickinson E Rehabilitation for older people: at risk in the new NHS. *British Medical Journal* 1998; **316**:1108–9.

2 Robinson J & Batstone G *Rehabilitation: a development challenge.* King's Fund, London 1996.

3 Tinetti ME, Speechley M, & Ginter SF Risk factors for falls among elderly persons living in the community. *New England Journal of Medicine* 1988; **319**:1701–7.

4 OPCS *1991 Mortality Statistics: cause, England & Wales.* HMSO, London 1993.

5 Colledge N Falls. *Reviews in Clinical Gerontology* 1997; 7:309–15.

6 van Weel C, Vermeulen H, & van den Bosch W Falls: a community care perspective. *Lancet* 1995; 345:1549–51.

7 Tinetti ME, Mendes de Leon CF, Doucette JT, *et al.* Fear of falling and fall-related efficacy in relation to functioning among community living elders *Journal of Gerontology* 1994; 49:140–7.

8 Alexander NB Postural control in older adults. *Journal of the American Geriatricians Society* 1994; 42:93–108.

9 Tallis R Rehabilitation of the elderly in the 21st century. *Journal of the Royal College of Physicians* 1992; 26(4):413–22.

10 Ried LD, Johnson RE, & Gettman DA Benzodiazepine exposure and functional status in older people. *Journal of the American Geriatricians Society* 1998; 46:71–6.

11 Iliffe S, Haines, AP, Gallivan S, *et al.* Alcohol consumption by elderly people: a general practice survey. *Age & Ageing* 1991; 20(2):120–3.

12 Chapuy MC, Arlot ME, & Dubouef F Vitamin D$_3$ and calcium to prevent hip fractures in elderly women. *New England Journal of Medicine* 1994; 331:821–7.

13 Egger G & Swinburn B An ecological approach to the obesity pandemic. *British Medical Journal* 1997; 315:477–80.

14 van Staveren WA, Burena J, De Groot L, *et al.* Dietary intakes in the elderly. *Facts & Research in Gerontology* 1992; 5:229–36.

15 Vellas B, Albarede JL, & Garry PJ Disease and aging: patterns of morbidity with age; relationship between aging & age-associated diseases. *American Journal of Clinical Nutrition* 1992; 55:S1225–S30.

16 McWhirter JP & Pennington CR Incidence and recognition of malnutrition in hospital. *British Medical Journal* 1994; 308:945–8.

17 Payette H Nutritional status of community-residing elderly with functional limitations. *Age and Nutrition* 1994; 5:4–5.

18 Thomas DR Outcome from protein–energy malnutrition in nursing home residents. *Facts & Research in gerontology* (supplement on Nutrition & Ageing). Springer, New York 1994.

19 Sullivan DH & Walls RC Impact of nutritional status on morbidity in a population of geriatric rehabilitation patients. *Journal of the American Geriatricians Society* 1994; 42:471–7.

20 Nutrition Screening Initiative *Report of nutrition screening, 1: Towards a common view.* American Academy of Family Physicians, American Dietetic Association, National Council on Ageing, Washington 1991.

21 Lee RD & Nieman DC *Nutritional assessment.* Brown & benchmark Publishers, Wisconsin 1993.

22 Verbrugge LM & Jette AM The disablement process. *Social Science and Medicine* 1994; **38**(1):1–14.

23 Nevitt MC, Cummings SR, Kidd S, *et al.* Risk factors for recurrent non-syncopal falls: a prospective study. *Journal of the American Medical Association* 1989; **261**:2663–8.

24 Hoenig H, Nusbaum JD, & Brummel-Smith K Geriatric rehabilitation: state of the art. *Journal of the American Geriatricians Society* 1997; **45**:1371–81.

25 Hu MH & Woollacott MH Balance evaluation, training and rehabilitation of frail fallers. *Reviews in Clinical Gerontology* 1996; **6**:85–99.

26 Gillespie LD, Gillespie WJ, Cumming R, *et al.* *Interventions to reduce the incidence of falling in the elderly.* Cochrane Library, The Cochrane Collaboration, Issue 4. Update Software,Oxford 1997.

27 Ebrahim S, Thompson PW, Baskaran V, *et al.* Randomised placebo-controlled trial of brisk walking in the promotion of post-menopausal osteoporosis. *Age & Ageing* 1997; **26**:253–60.

28 Feder G *Guidelines for the prevention of falls in older people.* Dept. of General Practice & Primary Care, Queen Mary & Westfield College, London 1998.

29 Mulrow CD, Gerety MB, Kanten D, *et al.* A randomised controlled trial of physical rehabilitation for very frail nursing home residents. *Journal of the American Medical Association* 1994; **271**:519–24.

30 Strawbridge WJ, Kaplan GA, Camacho BA, *et al.* The dynamics of disability and functional change in an elderly cohort: results from the Alameda County study. *Journal of the American Geriatricians Society* 1992; **40**:799-806.

31 Cambell AJ & Buchner DM Unstable disability and the fluctuations of frailty. *Age & Ageing* 1997; **26**(4): 315–8.

32 Dyer CAE, Watkins C, Gould C, *et al.* Risk factor assessment for falls: from a written check-list to the penless clinic. *Age & Ageing* 1998; **27**:569–72.

33 Robine JM & Ritchie K Healthy life expectancy: an evaluation of global indicators of change in population health. *British Medical Journal* 1991; **302**:457–60.

34 Kempen GIJ, Verbrugge LM, Merrill SS, *et al.* The impact of multiple impairments on disability in community-dwelling older people. *Age & Ageing* 1998; **27**:595–604.

35 Schulz R, Heckenhausen J, & Locher J Adult development, control and adaptive functioning. *Journal of Social Issues* 1991; **47**:177–96.

36 Heckhausen J & Schultz R Optimisation by selection and compensation: balancing primary and secondary control in life span development. *International Journal of Behavioral Development* 1993; **16**:287–303.

37 Taylor SE Adjustment to threatening events. *American Psychologist* 1983; **38**: 1161–73.

38 Schulz R & Williamson GM Psychosocial and behavioural dimensions of physical frailty *Journal Gerontology* 1993;**48**:39–43.

39 Tennant A, Fear J, Pickering A, *et al.* Prevalence of knee problems in the population aged 55 years and over: identifying the need for knee arthroplasty. *British Medical Journal* 1995;**310**:1291–3

40 Bowling A, Farquar M, & Grundy E Associations with changes in level of functional ability: results from a follow-up survey at two and a half years of people aged 85 years and over at baseline. *Ageing & Society* 1994;**14**:53-73

CHAPTER SIX

Vision and hearing problems in later life

Visual impairment

Visual impairment is common amongst older people and increases with advancing age. In community-based surveys of older people undertaken in the United Kingdom, visual acuity of less than 6/12 has been found in around 2% of subjects aged 65–74, and around 20% of subjects aged 75 and over.[1] This level of visual acuity is below the UK driving requirements. Larger surveys have been performed in the United States, and similar trends are seen there.[2]

Cataract and age-related macular degeneration (AMD) are the commonest causes of this visual loss, producing 63% and 20% of loss respectively in people aged 65 and over in a UK community survey.[1] Macular degeneration, with its bilateral clouding of central vision, is a particularly disabling impairment, affecting nearly one in five of those aged 85 or more.[3] Glaucoma is relatively uncommon, occuring in 7% of people in the same survey, but is the leading cause of acquired blindness.[4] Refraction defects are also very common, and are uncorrected or inadequately corrected in a quarter of those aged 65 and over and in almost half of those aged 75 and over.[5]

A number of adverse outcomes are associated with visual impairment, including:

- reduced functional ability and quality of life
- social isolation and loneliness
- falls and accidents (including road traffic accidents)
- depression, such that depressed patients are more functionally disabled by any given reduction in visual acuity
- an increased risk and increased severity of Alzheimer's disease.

Sudden or severe loss of vision can be an overwhelming personal and family catastrophe, affecting the patient's mobility, work, and personal relationships, yet if the change in eyesight is slow it is easier for others to underestimate the extent of its impact.[6] This list of associations makes screening for eye disease in older people in general practice a tempting option, but primary care workers should be cautious before embarking on any such project. The pattern of morbidity in later life can be complex, and causal effects cannot be attributed to associations, however strong they may seem. For example, visual problems are associated with general ill health, which could explain the association of visual impairment with falls. Although there is evidence that visual acuity, reduced visual field, impaired contrast sensitivity, and the presence of cataract may all combine to increase the risk of falls,[7] a recent systematic review found no evidence to support visual screening as a method of reducing this risk.[8]

Before a screening programme for eye disease is implemented primary care workers should be satisfied that the criteria for effectiveness of screening are met, as shown in Box 6.1.[9]

Box 6.1 *Criteria for evaluating the effectiveness of screening programmes*[9]

- Does the burden of suffering warrant suffering?
- Is there a good screening test?
- Are effective treatments or preventive measures available?
- Will those at risk accept screening?
- Do patients with positive screening results accept interventions and advice?
- Can the health service manage the consequences of the screening effort?

Assessing visual function

The first criterion is met, for the burden of eye disease seems very great and much of it may not be known. Half of those with visual impairment in the community study cited above[1] were not known to have eye disease by their general practitioners. Can the different causes of visual loss be detected reliably, easily, and cheaply in community settings? If they can, primary care teams may have the potential to improve the quality of everyday life for many older patients, reduce their risk of recurrent falls, diminish the number of injuries experienced by older people in road accidents, and reduce the social isolation and loneliness of vulnerable individuals.

This task is a complex one because visual function appears to be more important in determining the risk of an adverse event than any particular change in the performance of the eyes. For example, visual acuity, as measured by a Snellen chart, may not correlate with visual function because some individuals with very poor acuity may deny that they have any visual problem at all. Nor is loss of visual acuity always associated with increased risk of recurrent falls, hip fractures, or road accidents.[7] The difficulties in identifying those older people in the community most at risk through visual impairment become evident when we investigate the relationships between vision and driving accidents.

The crash rate per driver amongst those aged 65 and over is low, probably because older drivers tend to drive shorter distances and avoid driving at night, in heavy traffic, or in bad weather. However, the crash rate per mile driven for older drivers is higher than that for younger adults, and is lower than only one other group, teenagers. Right-of-way and turning accidents occur particularly frequently with older drivers, and may be due to age-related changes in vision that cause problems with:[10]

- merging traffic streams
- vehicles appearing unexpectedly in their peripheral vision
- judging own speed and that of approaching vehicles
- reading poorly lit road signs or dim vehicle information displays.

It is not clear how these problems can be overcome or ameliorated, and the tendency of many older people is to avoid driving in situations that put them at most risk. This may not be practical for some, especially if they do have a significant social role in collecting children from school, working for voluntary bodies, or even in maintaining paid employment. The increase in the pace and density of modern traffic puts older drivers at a disadvantage, although this may diminish as a generation who learned to drive late in life gives way to one which grew up in an automotive society.[11] In the meantime we need pragmatic approaches for detecting and assessing the older driver with functional deficits, perhaps by measuring a combination of visual ability and higher order attentional skills through 'useful field of view' (UFOV) tests.[12]

The same complexity applies to falls where contrast sensitivity, visual field size, and visual acuity appear to be implicated in recurrent falling,[7] possibly through their impact on posture stabilization. How can the primary care team begin to identify those at risk from such complex impairments? How and why vision should be assessed were not specified in the 1990 GP contract. The Royal College of General Practitioners' interpretation of the 1990 contract was to include in the 75-and-over check a simple question about visual function to identify unreported problems. Specific screening procedures for glaucoma or diabetic retinopathy have not been included in the over-75 programme (nor in trials of multiphasic screening) despite the impact of these problems on visual function, and the treatments available for them.

Screening tests

Screening questions of the kind advocated by the Royal College of General Practitioners are poor at detecting clinically significant reductions in visual acuity, as Table 6.1 shows.

The middle question appears to be more sensitive than the others, but it was asked of people who had already identified themselves as having some kind of visual problem. By combining the questions the sensitivity of identifying visual acuity of <6/12 increases to 86%.

Testing distance acuity with a Snellen chart is quick and easy, and 95% of GPs have such charts. The test is not reliable if not used at the correct distance and in poor illumination, and will not detect uncorrected presbyopia, for which reading charts are needed. Pinhole testing with the Snellen chart can

Table 6.1 *Screening questions of the kind advocated by the Royal College of General Practitioners (derived from Smeeth 1998)*[13]

Question	Visual Acuity Comparison	Sensitivity	Specificity
Do you have difficulty seeing distant objects with spectacles if you have them?	<6/18	28%	93%
Are you able to recognize a friend across the road?	<6/18	64%	48%
Two questions: Have you ever worn glasses or contact lenses? Followed by: Do you have trouble with your vision even when wearing glasses or contact lenses?	Between 6/12 & 6/18	34%	84%

help distinguish refractive from non-refractive visual impairment. Looking for a red reflex using an ophthalmoscope is also easy and brief, and can be used to identify individuals with cataracts.

Who should have their vision assessed in primary care, and by whom? The lack of evidence of benefit from screening asymptomatic older people means that a whole-population approach cannot be recommended.[13] Those who present with symptoms should be assessed, using a combination of questions, a check for a red reflex, and acuity measurement with use of a pin-hole in the impaired. Three-quarters of older people who fall and are admitted to hospital are likely to have remediable visual defects,[14] and so this group (in fact, any recurrent fallers) should be assessed. Although it is not clear what level of visual acuity should act as a threshold for referral for specialist review, any symptoms apparently impairing daily life, or putting the individual at risk, should be investigated further.

The effectiveness of treatment

Assessment of visual function in primary care may be difficult, but intervention seems effective across a broad range of visual problems once patients are identified. Improvement in visual function after diagnosis of cataract or degenerative eye disease is followed by improvement in home and social activities, quality of life and satisfaction, mental health, and even driving ability by day or night – regardless of condition or treatment.[15] Cataract surgery is particularly effective in improving the patient's quality of life, and attention to lighting, visual aids, adaptive equipment, and patient education can all help to lessen the impact of visual disability.[5]

The effectiveness of treatment of age-related macular degeneration is as yet unknown, the treatment (with argon laser photocoagulation) for some forms of AMD being still experimental, so screening with Amsler grids to detect early central distortion of vision is probably inappropriate. However, AMD may be amenable to prevention in ways that other eye diseases are not because it appears to be linked to atherosclerosis[16] and so may be reduced if cardiovascular disease (CVD) risk factors are controlled. Similarly, moderate wine consumption may have a protective effect against AMD (as it apparently does for CVD) through antioxidant effects and reduced platelet aggregation,[17] whilst beer has the opposite impact,[18] perhaps because of its pro-oxidant effect. Primary care research networks could do worse than evaluate the impact of CVD risk factor modification and lifestyle changes in general practice populations on the incidence and prevalence of macular degeneration.

Acceptance of interventions

In the 1970s 40% of visually impaired people identified in a community survey had never seen an ophthalmologist, and the Office of Population Censuses and Surveys (OPCS) disability survey of 1988 estimated that twice as many people are visually impaired as can be accounted for by those registered blind or partially sighted.[1] Visual problems in older people may go unreported and unrecognized for a number of reasons, including:

- decreased patient expectation in old age
- a belief that nothing can be done to help
- failure by the patient to recognize their visual loss
- the presence of another handicap which dominates the perception of difficulties
- fears about treatment such as surgery
- costs of testing or treatment
- the stigma of blindness.

We should not forget that sensory defects disable all who come into contact with them, including doctors, who may lose part of their ability to communicate sensitively and empathically with a visually impaired patient. We may give up trying to communicate, avoid or minimize contact, and inadvertently indicate that the partially sighted person should stop troubling us. Not surprisingly, older people with significant visual (or hearing) losses perceive themselves as a burden to others[6].

Reactions to failing vision can include the following stages:

- disbelief and denial
- pining for lost function, with preoccupation with the visual past, anxiety symptoms, and emotional lability, irritability, and anger
- subsequent depression
- resolution, sometimes related to events such as preparing a meal which demonstrate self-sufficiency and increase self-esteem.

Extreme loss of vision may be associated with persistent denial of blindness, with unrealistic hopes of recovery and refusal to learn new, appropriate skills, pursuit of unrealistic treatment options, and a desire for more investigations and specialist assessments. Given the potential for grief at loss of visual function, it is hardly surprising that one in three older people identified as visually impaired in a community survey did not take up the specialist assessment offered to them.[5]

Provision of specialist treatment

Effective treatment is available for many symptomatic older patients with visual problems, for example cataract surgery, but waiting lists are sometimes long. Should visual assessment be done by more skilled professionals than general practitioners, given the apparent tendency of GPs to delay referral for glaucoma, and our lack of accuracy in identifying retinopathy, even after training? If opticians and optometrists are to play a role in early detection of remediable eye disease, do charges for providing spectacles, and previously for testing, act as obstacles in a population where one-third survive on a low income? Answering these questions is important, given the likely rise in demand for treatment of eye diseases as the population continues to age. For example, the demand for specialist investigation and treatment of open angle glaucoma, cataract, and age-related macular degeneration increases three, four, and eight times respectively between the age groups 60–69 and 80 and over.[19] suggesting that the expected 16% increase in the 80-and-over population is likely to have a significant impact on specialist eye services. Referral thresholds may also fall, as they did following the introduction of intra-ocular lens implantation, exerting more pressure on services.

We can summarise the issues facing primary care workers this way:
Practitioners should:

- focus assessment of vision on older patients with symptomatic eye disease and on those who fall repeatedly using a combination of questions, visual acuity measurement, pinhole testing, and red reflex testing
- liaise closely with local opticians and optometrists before referring for specialist review
- follow up with support for those found to be profoundly visually impaired.

Primary care groups should:

- consider the level of extra investment needed in their locality for specialist eye services for older people
- establish minimum standards for assessment of eye problems, and support them with appropriate training
- review the information made available for older patients with visual impairment about their condition and possible treatments or responses.

Primary care research networks could consider:

- how best to assess visual fitness to drive in later life
- measuring the impact of improving visual function on the incidence of falls
- studying the effect pf cardiovascular risk factor control on AMD incidence, prevalance, and severity.

Deafness

Mrs I. took great care to wear her hearing aid every day, even when she had no visitors, but rarely fitted the battery. The district nurse who was visiting her to dress her leg ulcer found this out, and asked her why she did this. Her reply was: 'If I wear the aid people stop going on at me about using it, and if I leave the batteries out I don't hear the horrible hissing.'

Mrs I. is not alone in any aspect of her problem. Deafness is a common problem of later life, but seemingly not as damaging to the individual as visual loss, so that remedial action is not taken as frequently and as effectively as it might be. Nevertheless there is a case for early detection and intervention, in primary care, which we will now explore.

About a quarter of individuals aged 65 and over report a problem with their hearing, and one-third have measurable hearing loss.[20] It is estimated that 8.7 million adults in Britain have some degree of deafness, of whom 75% are aged 65 or over.[21] A single process accounts for this common impairment, unlike visual loss, for the great majority have presbycusis, a gradual and progressive, bilateral, high-frequency sensorineural loss that impairs understanding of speech. Presbycusis is related to the physiological ageing process, but may be worsened by other medical conditions,[22] including:

- diabetes
- hypothyroidism
- hyperlipidaemia
- hypertension
- ischaemic heart disease
- stroke
- arthritis
- chronic lung disease
- renal disease
- viral and bacterial infections.

Behavioural and environmental factors such as alcohol consumption or noise exposure also seem to exacerbate presbycusis, and some drugs (aspirin, diuretics such as frusemide and bumetanide, and antibiotics) are implicated as causes. The mechanisms that produce these relationships between a wide range of disorders and hearing loss are unclear, and it is not known whether optimizing the management of, say, diabetes or chronic obstructive pulmonary disease (COPD) makes any difference to hearing function or the progress of presbycusis.

Whilst presbycusis accounts for the great majority of hearing loss in older people, it is not the only cause of hearing problems and symptoms, and needs to be distinguished from:

• conductive hearing loss sometimes due to ear infection, and rarely to tumours of the middle ear
• sensorineural loss, due to Ménière's disease or an acoustic neuroma.

Sudden onset of sensorineural deafness or unilateral symptoms warrant further investigation and referral to an ear, nose, and throat (ENT) clinic, whilst bilateral sensorineural loss uncomplicated by infection, fluctuation, persistent tinnitus, or vertigo may be best investigated in an audiology clinic, after an appropriate work-up (see below).

The criteria for screening which we applied earlier in this chapter to visual loss are met by hearing loss, up to a point. The burden of disease and disability is significant, there are brief screening tests, and interventions can be effective. However, patient concordance with screening and intervention is not great, and the health service is probably unable to cope with the volume of demand for assessment and remedial action. The more we investigate this, the more complex the problems appear, and the more we learn about the relationship between impairment and disability.

Clinical burden

Deafness is associated with a diminished sense of well-being, and adverse effects on physical, cognitive, emotional, behavioural, and social functioning.[20] Deaf older people report greater limitations in their activity compared with their peers with normal hearing, and make more demands on medical services.[23] There is also a suspicion that deafness increases the risks of major driving accidents.[24] The impact of hearing loss on older people seems sufficient to produce communication difficulties and social and sometimes emotional isolation, although this withdrawal may be accepted as the 'least worst' option, as with Mrs I. above, and be accepted by others as a normal adaptation to ageing. Deafness may contribute to the onset of depression, and to the development of cognitive impairment,[20] although these are not consistent findings, and depressed and cognitively impaired individuals are more likely to report hearing impairment that is not detectable on objective examination.[22] The risks of deafness are higher in working-class populations, probably because of occupational noise exposure or exposure to organic toxic solvents.[22] However, although the burden of deafness appears to be significant for older people, it lacks the persuasive power of visual loss because it does not impact forcefully on services, and produces changes in behaviour that can be attributed to 'old age'.

Screening tests

As with visual loss, no single, brief screening instrument is sensitive or specific enough to be used routinely in population screening. A combination of two approaches performs better, and is justifiable in a case-finding approach after clinical suspicion has been aroused. Whisper tests, the finger-rub test, and use of a tuning fork are not reliable alone, although they may have some value in the first stage of an assessment in alerting the clinician to the potential for deafness in the patient. An audiometry examination, or use of an audioscope, is appropriate given that the latter's sensitivity in detecting failure to hear a 40 dB tone ranges from 87% to 96%, with specificities of 70% to 90%, and good repeatability.[20]

A self-assessment questionnaire is a useful adjunct to audiometry, the most extensively tested and widely used being the Hearing Handicap Inventory for the Elderly (screening version) Box 6.2.[25]

Box 6.2 *Hearing Handicap Inventory for the Elderly (screening version)*

- Does a hearing problem cause you to feel embarassed when you meet new people?
- Does a hearing problem cause you to feel frustrated when talking to members of your family?
- Do you have difficulties hearing when someone talks in a whisper?
- Do you feel handicapped by a hearing problem?
- Does a hearing problem cause you difficulty when visiting friends, relatives, or neighbours?
- Does a hearing problem cause you to attend religious services less often than you would like?
- Does a hearing problem cause you to have arguments with family members?
- Does a hearing problem cause you to have difficulty when listening to the television or radio?
- Do you feel that any difficulty with your hearing limits/hampers your personal or social life?
- Does a hearing problem cause you difficulty when in a restaurant with family or friends?

A 'no' response scores zero, 'sometimes' scores 2, and 'yes' scores 4. A score of less than 10 indicates no handicap, and greater than 24 indicates moderate to severe handicap. Although religious belief and church attendance are still important in some older cohorts in the UK, the question on attendance at religious services (derived from American social habits) may need modification for British populations.

Effective interventions and patient concordance

There are no randomized controlled trials of interventions in the community to guide practitioners about the effectiveness of treatments, but before-and-after and case–control community studies and RCTs in selected populations have demonstrated improved psychological and social functioning, better communication, and fewer depression symptoms after hearing-aid fitting.[20]

Uptake of hearing aids depends on their cost to the patient, and their capacity to induce embarrassment by drawing attention to the handicap, whilst actual use may be determined by adverse effects such as significant amplification of background noise.

According to one American community study, about one in five of those who might benefit from sound amplification use or have tried hearing aids, with greatest use among those with greatest disability and the most educated,[26] but it does not seem possible as yet to identify those who are most likely to take up and use remediable services. Adapting to hearing-aid use does not appear easy for many older people, making correct fitting, training in listening strategies and communication techniques, and continuing support and counselling essential, even if new digital and programmable technologies make aids easier to use.[27]

Service implications

If there are five million people aged 65 and over with significant hearing impairment due to presbycusis, and only one million use or have tried hearing aids, how can the NHS reach the other four million without overloading audiology services and citizens' private budgets? The cost of hearing aids appears to be a barrier to uptake, so an optimal programme would need to fund both the diagnostic service and the supply and maintainance of aids. Primary care group boards can calculate the likely cost of such a service as a salutary exercise in meeting unmet need.

We can summarize the implications of hearing loss like this:
Practitioners should:

- respond to clinical suspicion of deafness in older patients with a self-completion questionnaire like the Hearing Handicap Inventory for the elderly (screening version), followed by audiometry/audioscope assessment
- use simple tests to identify conductive disorders, supplementing a history that includes noise exposure and drug use
- refer to audiology or ENT according to findings with follow-up and support of hearing-aid users.

Primary Care Groups should:

- ensure that appropriate training programmes are in place for primary care workers, to enhance identification of hearing impairment
- consider support for self-help initiatives for deaf older patients
- calculate the likely cost of comprehensive local diagnostic, remedial, and support services for hearing impairment.

Primary care research networks should:

- identify those who are most likely to act on their perceived impairment to allow targeting of resources
- carry out a randomized controlled trial of interventions to reduce hearing impairment in the community – it remains to be done!

References

1 Wormald RP, Wright LA, Courtney P, *et al.* Visual problems in the elderly population and implications for services. *British Medical Journal* 1992; **304**:1226–9.

2 Klein R, Klein BE, Linton KL, *et al.* The Beaver Dam eye study: visual acuity. *Ophthalmology* 1991; **98**:1310–15.

3 Mitchell P, Smith W, Attebo K, *et al.* Prevalence of age-related maculopathy in Australia: the Blue Mountains Eye Study. *Ophthalmology* 1995; **102**(10): 1450–60.

4 Evans JR *Causes of blindness and partial sight in England & Wales 1990–91.* Studies on Medical and Population Subjects, Report 57. HMSO, London 1995.

5 Smeeth L Screening older people for impaired vision. *Family Practice* 1998; **15**:S24–S29.

6 Fitzgerald R & Murray Parker C Blindness and loss of other sensory and cognitive functions. *British Medical Journal* 1998; **316**:1160–3.

7 Ivers RQ, Cumming RG, Mitchell P, *et al.* Visual impairment and falls in older adults: the Blue Mountains eye study. *Journal of the American Geriatricians Society;* 1998: **46**:58–64.

8 NHS Centre for Reviews & Disemination, University of York Preventing falls and subsequent injury in older people. *Effective Health Care* 1996; **2**:4.

9 Cadman D, Chambers L, Feldman W, *et al.* Assessing the effectiveness of community screening programs. *Journal of the American Medical Association* 1984; **251**:1580–5.

10 Waller JA Health status and motor vehicle crashes. *New England Journal of Medicine* 1991; **324**:54–5.

11 Kline DW, Kline TJB, Fozard JL, *et al.* Vision, ageing and driving: the problems of older drivers. *Journal of Gerontology* 1992; **47**:27–34.

12 Owsley C Vision and driving in the elderly. *Optometry & Vision Science* 1994; **71**(12):727–35.

13 Smeeth L & Iliffe S Effectiveness of screening older people for impaired vision in community settings: systematic review of evidence from randomised controlled trials. *British Medical Journal* 1998; **316**:660–3.

14 Jack CIA, Smith T, Neoh C, *et al.* Prevalence of low vision in elderly patients admitted to an acute geriatric unit in Liverpool: elderly people who fall are more likely to have low vision. *Gerontology* 1995; **41**:280–5.

15 Brenner MH, Curbow B, Javitt JC, *et al.* Vision change and quality of life in the elderly: response to cataract surgery and treatment of other chronic ocular conditions *Archives of Ophthalmology* 1993; **111**(5):680–5.

16 Vingerling JR, Dielmans I, Bots ML, *et al.* Age-related macular degeneration is associated with atherosclerosis: The Rotterdam study. *American Journal of Epidemiology* 1995; **142**:404–9.

17 Obisesan TO, Hirsch R, Kosoko O, *et al.* Moderate wine consumption is associated with decreased odds of developing age-related macular degeneration in NHANES-1. *Journal of the American Geriatricians Society* 1998; **46**:1-7.

18 Ritter LL, Klein R, Klein BEK, *et al.* Alcohol use and age-related maculopathy in the Beaver Dam eye study. *American Journal of Ophthalmology* 1995; **120**:190–6.

19 Sheldrick J, Vernon SA, Wilson A, *et al.* Demand incidence and episode rates of ophthalmic disease in a defined urban population. *British Medical Journal* 1992; **305**:933–6.

20 Mulrow CD & Lichtenstein MJ Screening for hearing impairment in the elderly: rationale and strategy. J. Gen. Intern. Med. 1991; **6**:249–58.

21 Roper TA & Setchfield N Diagnosis and management of impaired hearing. *Geriatric Medicine* 1998; **November:**49–52.

22 Maggi S, Minicuci N, Martini A, *et al.* Prevalence rates of hearing impairment and co-morbid conditions in older people: the Veneto study. *Journal of the American Geriatricians Society* 1998; **46**:1069–74.

23 Hearing ability of persons by socio-economic characteristics. PHS82-1568:8-20. Dept of Health & Human Services, United States 1982.

24 McCloskey LW, Koepsell TD, Wolf ME *et al.* Motor vehicle collision injuries and sensory impairments of older drivers. *Age & Ageing* 1994; **23**(4):267–73.

25 Lichtenstein MJ, Bess FH, & Logan SA Diagnostic performance of the Hearing Handicap Inventory for the Elderly (screening version) against different definitions of hearing loss. *Ear Hear* 1988; **9**:208–11.

26 Popelka MM, Cruikshanks KJ, Wiley TL, *et al.* Low prevalence of hearing-aid use among older adults with hearing loss: the epidemiology of hearing loss study. *Journal of the American Geriatricians Society* 1998; **46**:1075–8.

27 Miller ST & Zapala DA Better use of hearing aids in hearing-impaired adults. *Journal of the American Geriatricians Society* 1998; **46**:1168–9.

CHAPTER SEVEN

Cardiovascular disease and stroke

There are four target areas in cardiovascular disease as it affects older people where the evidence base for intervention is good enough to warrant a systematic approach to case-finding and case management. They are:

(1) **identifying all individuals with left ventricular failure and initiating ACE inhibitor therapy**. The evidence supporting the use of ACE inhibitors in reducing mortality and morbidity from ventricular failure is good, with reduction in hospital admissions. Ventricular failure is over-diagnosed clinically and requires echocardiography for reliable diagnosis. Reducing the mortality from stroke and myocardial infarctions (MIs) through better blood pressure control may increase the number of patients entering this diagnostic group (see below).

(2) **treating hypertension in older people**. The number with hypertension who must be treated to avoid one cardiovascular event falls with advancing age, at least up to 75 years, but there appear to be age barriers to the initiation of treatment. If these can be overcome, in part through implementing an audit cycle and systematic case management in practices, the rate of strokes and infarcts will decrease, although perhaps at the expense of a rise in the prevalence of ventricular failure.

(3) **using warfarin or aspirin for the prevention of stroke in individuals with chronic atrial fibrillation** (AF). Warfarin reduces the risk of stroke in patients with AF by 68%; aspirin has a smaller effect. A risk stratification approach can help balance risks and benefits of treatment with these drugs, both of which are underprescribed in the 6% of the population over 65 who have AF.

(4) **using aspirin in secondary prevention of cardiovascular disease**. Aspirin reduces the risk of further cardiovascular events in 20% of patients who have angina, past infarction, transient ischaemic attacks (TIAs), and stroke, but is underprescribed. Given the size of this population, the potential gains from a systematic approach to their care are great.

Other issues – for example, smoking cessation programmes and exercise promotion – are important and should be further researched, precisely

135

because the evidence supporting their effectiveness in primary care settings is less compelling.

Heart failure

Congestive heart failure affects 3–5% of the population aged 65 and over, and its incidence and prevalence double with each advancing decade.[1] A GP with a list of 2000 and 'average' demography will see 10 new cases of heart failure a year, and have another 10 established cases.[2] Between four and five of those with established heart failure will be admitted to hospital each year, and up to 60% of those with severe heart failure will die each year. For both the patient and the primary care team congestive heart failure is a common, disabling, progressive, and serious illness. Fortunately, once diagnosed it is more amenable to medical intervention than many common, disabling disorders of later life, so that practitioners can produce significant gains for their patients by simply applying current knowledge. Congestive heart failure (CHF) is a syndrome in which the heart fails to maintain an adequate output, resulting in underperfusion and lowered blood pressure, with consequent triggering of the renin–angiotensin system. This increases heart rate, peripheral resistance, and myocardial contractility, which are beneficial in the short term but which become harmful if sustained. Treatment consists essentially of interfering with the renin-angiotensin system, and reducing sympathetic drive, although the underlying pathophysiology is still not fully understood.[3]

Diagnosis of CHF can be difficult because physical signs may be minimal in early but symptomatic stages of the disease process, or misleading, especially when the concurrent symptoms of co-morbidity (for example, COPD) distort the clinical picture. About half of all patients with CHF are not diagnosed, and about half of those diagnosed as having CHF by clinical examination alone have the diagnosis confirmed on echocardiography.

Investigation of CHF hinges on echocardiography, which is a quick, cheap, and reliable method for studying systolic and diastolic function, and identifying left ventricular hypertrophy and valvular disease. Echocardiography performs better as a diagnostic tool for CHF than a plain chest x-ray, which is a specific but not very sensitive test, especially in mild or compensated failure, and is sometimes difficult to interpret when pulmonary disease or kyphoscoliosis complicate the picture. A 12-lead electrocardiogram (ECG) can help to reach the diagnosis, but is sensitive to CHF rather than specific for heart failure due to systolic dysfunction, and is less useful than echocardiography in providing the baseline information needed to target therapy appropriately. Only a third of patients receiving treatment for heart failure have an echocardiogram, partly because of diagnoses reached and decisions taken by GPs, and partly through lack of resources. Use of x-rays and 12-lead ECGs may therefore be a necessary 'second best' approach to diagnosis, as shown in Figure 7.1

Practitioners will need access to echocardiography, either through specialist cardiology access or by direct access, or even through deployment of

Figure 7.1 Investigation of congestive heart failure in primary care (modified from the North of England Guidelines, 1998).

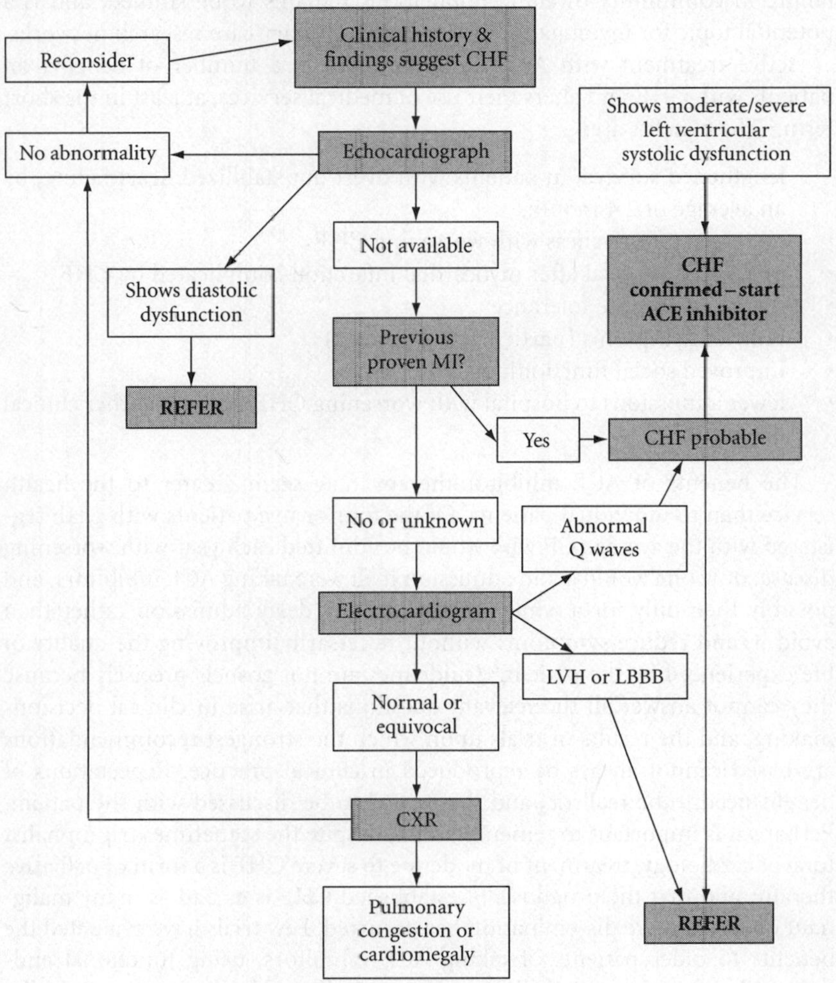

Clinical history & findings suggest CHF

Reconsider

No abnormality

Echocardiograph

Shows moderate/severe left ventricular systolic dysfunction

Not available

CHF confirmed – start ACE inhibitor

Shows diastolic dysfunction

REFER

Previous proven MI?

Yes → CHF probable

No or unknown

Abnormal Q waves

Electrocardiogram

LVH or LBBB

Normal or equivocal

CXR

Pulmonary congestion or cardiomegaly

REFER

portable echocardiography in the community. Since there is evidence that diagnosis and active treatment is cost-effective, the factor limiting the spread of echocardiography services is likely to be the availability of trained technicians.

Diastolic dysfunction and left ventricular hypertrophy (LVH) without ventricular dysfunction, often associated with hypertension, need to be identified because the implications for treatment can be different. For example, there is no evidence that ACE inhibitors are useful in treating diastolic dysfunction, and vasodilators may be hazardous, so specialist assessment is important in reviewing other treatments (see below).

Natriuretic peptides produced by the atrial and ventricular myocardium are potentially useful markers of heart failure,[4] whilst brain natriuretic peptide levels in blood have prognostic significance for older patients with or without clinical features of CHF.[5] Their use in identification and management of heart failure in community-dwelling populations remains to be studied, and is a potential topic for investigation by emerging primary care research networks.

Active treatment with ACE inhibitors confers a number of benefits on patients with CHF, and alters their use of medical services, at least in the short term.[2] The benefits are:

- lengthened survival in patients with overt but stabilized heart failure, by an average of 2.4 months
- increased effectiveness with worsening CHF
- prolonged survival after myocardial infarction complicated by CHF
- increased exercise tolerance
- reduced symptoms (particularly dyspnoea)
- improved social functioning
- fewer admissions to hospital with worsening CHF, and with other clinical diagnoses.

The benefits of ACE inhibitor therapy may seem greater to the health service than to individual patients. Of the four or five patients with CHF registered with the average GP who would be admitted each year with worsening disease, only one would avoid admission if all were taking ACE inhibitors, and possibly then only for a while. Treatment may delay admission rather than avoid it, and reduce symptoms without necessarily improving the quality of life experienced by the patient.[6] Guidelines are not gospels precisely because they cannot answer all the relevant questions that arise in clinical decision-making, and the results of trials upon which the strongest recommendations are based cannot always be reproduced in clinical practice. Expectations of benefit need to be realistic, and these need to be discussed with the patient. Perhaps it is important to remember that, despite the sometimes triumphalist tone of cardiology, treatment of moderate to severe CHF is a form of palliative therapy, and that the prognosis of established CHF is as bad as many malignant diseases where dissemination has occurred. Few trials have evaluated the benefits to older patients of taking ACE inhibitors, using functional endpoints like activities of daily living or timed walking,[7] but reducing morbidity substantially may be more important for individuals than reducing mortality rates by postponing death until after the study period.

Mrs J. (aged 78) had had her hypertension well controlled on thiazide diuretics alone for over a decade, but during the previous winter she had become increasingly breathless on exertion, and the dependency that had slowly increased over the last few years became much worse. Her blood pressure control also worsened, although she showed no change in her pattern of medication use, and had no change in cognitive functioning on testing with the Mini-Mental State Examination. Her GP suggested to her that she should start using an ACE inhibitor to control both her rising blood pressure and her apparent CHF, and she reluctantly agreed to this after lengthy discussion with her 63-year-old daughter.

She was admitted to the community ward of the local hospital, under her

GP's care, where the protocol for ACE inhibitor introduction was followed by the nursing staff (see below). Her chest X-ray and ECG showed changes suggestive of CHF, so an echocardiogram was not performed She experienced no adverse effects with a small dose of enalapril, and this was increased to 10 mg before discharge, and 20 mg daily at home, with reintroduction of a lower dose of thiazide diuretic after some weeks.

Her oedema did diminish, but very slowly, and it never returned to what both she and her GP felt was 'normal'. Her exertional dyspnoea decreased within a few days, and she was able to climb her stairs easily, get from her first floor flat into her garden, and go shopping with her daughter once a week. These changes were welcome, but she said that she never felt 'right' and that her tiredness was not altered by the new medication. She was not convinced that she should continue to take it, but understood that her breathlessness might suddenly worsen if she stopped.

Hyperkalaemia and hypotension are hazards of treatment with ACE inhibitors, and both initiation and continuation of treatment should take these risks into account. Recommendations for initiating treatment derived from both the North of England Guidelines and the US Agency for Health Care Policy and Research are shown in Box 7.1.

Box 7.1 *Recommendations for initiating ACE inhibitor treatment in older patients*

1. Check blood pressure and creatinine and electrolytes.
2. Cease treatment with potassium-sparing diuretics, and only restore them if the patient remains hypokalaemic on ACE inhibitors.
3. Withhold thiazide diuretics for at least 24 hours to allow resolution of volume depletion.
4. Initiation of ACE inhibitor treatment should take place in hospital if:
   - sodium concentration <135 mmoles/1
   - creatinine concentration is >150 mmoles/1
   - systolic BP is <100
   - more than 80 mg frusemide is needed daily to control symptoms
   - symptoms of heart failure are severe.
5. Use lower starting doses with advancing age, and titrate upwards over 2–3 weeks, aiming to reach doses used in trials, whilst informing the patient about adverse effects.
6. Use with caution in patients with peripheral vascular disease because of the risk of renal artery stenosis and renal failure.
7. Monitor, as in 1, until the effective therapeutic dose is reached, and then at least annually.

What can be done if an older patient who fits the criteria for treatment with ACE inhibitors is unable to take any of the available preparations because of adverse effects? There are a small number of alternatives which should be considered:

- Diuretics relieve dyspnoea and oedema by correcting salt and water over-load, but have no impact on left ventricular function, and may impair the quality of life. They can be used with ACE inhibitors, subject to the provisos noted above.
- Digoxin does reduce the rate of hospital admission for CHF, but has no effect on overall mortality, and its use in older people with CHF who are in sinus rhythm remains controversial.
- Hydralazine and isosorbide dinitrate in combination improve both symptoms and survival in CHF.
- Angiotensin receptor antagonists such as losartan may become important forms of therapy, since they may lack some of the adverse effects of ACE inhibitors whilst having a dramatic effect on mortality rates in older patients with CHF.[8]

Diastolic dysfunction needs to be mentioned because its early diagnosis by echocardiography places the patient firmly in the realm of specialist care, at least for the time it takes for primary care teams to master the systematic care of older people with congestive heart failure due to the commoner systolic dysfunction. Briefly, diuretics may worsen the symptoms of diastolic dysfunction by reducing intravascular volume and cardiac output, ACE inhibitors are of unproven benefit, and the newer calcium antagonists like nisoldipine appear to have beneficial effects on diastolic ventricular function.

Key messages for practitioners, primary care groups, and research networks are:

For practitioners:

- all clinical diagnoses of CHF should be reviewed using echocardiography as the diagnostic tool of choice
- ACE inhibitors should be used in CHF due to left ventricular systolic dysfunction, with careful attention to guidelines on introduction and maintenance of therapy
- reframing CHF management as a form of palliative therapy may emphasize the need to inform patients and their families about the condition and its treatments.

For primary care groups:

- echocardiography services may need to be developed, and this appears to be justified on cost-effectiveness grounds
- training for management of CHF in primary care might emphasize it as an example of palliative care
- specialist palliative care services could be extended to include patients dying from non-malignant disease like CHF
- audit of CHF management could usefully include both patient and professional perspectives on the quality of life during active treatment.

For primary care research networks:

- Is open-access echocardiography preferable to and cheaper than specialist cardiology services in the management of CHF?
- What are the best strategies for initiating ACE inhibitor treatment in the community?
- What gains can be made in the quality of life of patients with CHF using different treatment approaches?

Hypertension

Older people with elevated blood pressure are at greater risk of both stroke and heart disease compared with younger people with the same level of pressure. Treatment of hypertension at all ages up to 80 reduces the incidence of, and mortality from, both heart disease and stroke, although general practitioners and practice nurses need to overcome a bias towards treating younger rather than older patients if these benefits are to be obtained.[9] The odds ratios for an adverse effect from hypertension fall with treatment to 0.75 for heart disease and 0.66 for stroke in those aged 65–80 years, and the number needed to treat to avoid one stroke death in younger hypertensives (under 65) is 365, compared with 193 people in the 65-and-over age group.[10] Hypertension is not identified adequately in Britain, with only 63% of those with pressures of 160/95 known to be hypertensive, only half of these treated, and only 30% achieving satisfactory blood pressure control. This compares unfavourably with results from the USA where 89% were detected, 79% treated, and 64% controlled.[11]

Blood pressure levels consistently elevated above 150/90 in patients up to 80 years of age warrant intervention, which should consist of the following elements.[12]

- reduction in salt consumption by avoiding salty foods, and not adding salt during cooking or at the table. This may reduce the stroke risk by up to 30%
- reducing the weight of obese patients (BMI of 30 or more), which together with salt reduction will lower stroke or cardiovascular event risk by 53%
- reducing alcohol consumption
- promoting smoking cessation
- encouraging brisk walking for 30 minutes a day, for three or four days per week, if possible, which has been shown to reduce blood pressure, at least up to 75 years of age
- using a thiazide diuretic as a first choice of antihypertensive, calcium antagonists as a second choice, and a beta-blocker as the third choice–all having been shown to be effective in lowering blood pressure and reducing stroke rates and cardiovascular events in older people.

The value of ACE inhibitors, angiotensin II inhibitors, and alpha-blockers in the treatment of hypertension in older people is not yet clear, but is likely to become so as current trials report in the next few years. How best to manage hypertension in patients aged 80 or more is also uncertain.

Atherosclerotic disease accounts for considerable cognitive impairment in older people in the community,[13] so one outcome of better control of hypertension and cardiovascular risk factors may be a subsequent reduction in the incidence of the vascular forms of dementia.

Concordance with medication

Reluctance to continue medication for hypertension control is common, with nearly 90% of patients reporting adverse effects from their medication and over 20 % stopping drug treatment without returning to their GP, in one recent study.[14] Adverse effects of antihypertensive medication in older people are sometimes misunderstood by practitioners (Box 7.2).

Box 7.2 *Adverse effects of antihypertensive medication in older people*

Thiazide diuretics:

*   do not often produce significant hypokalaemia and use of combination forms with potassium supplements is not usually indicated
*   can induce glucose intolerance, which may take years to develop
*   have little or no adverse effects on lipid profiles
*   are associated with reported impotence no more often than placebo.

Calcium channel antagonists:

*   cause flushing, dizziness, palpatations, and ankle oedema sufficient to prompt drug withdrawal in up to 30% of users.

Beta-blockers:

*   need to be avoided by patients with asthma, peripheral vascular disease, and Raynaud's phenomenon.

Cessation of treatment is possible in a small proportion of older hypertensives, especially if they are using low-dose monotherapy and have low blood pressure readings before withdrawal. Only 20% of those in whom medication withdrawal is tried will remain off hypertensive medication two years later.[15] Likewise, withdrawal of long-term diuretic treatment in older patients leads to increases in blood pressure to hypertensive values or symptoms of heart failure in most cases.[16] Not surprisingly, withdrawal of antihypertensive therapy in older people is seen as a dangerous experiment by some clinicians.[17]

Secondary prevention strategies

Health promotion in primary care has an unhappy history, with little evidence that community-based, multifactorial interventions make much impact on risk factors for cardiovascular disease, or on cardiovascular disease itself.[18] However, targeted interventions aiming for secondary prevention of cardio-vascular events look promising, with evidence that there is enough suboptimal treatment to justify the effort of case management,[19] and that this management rapidly produces improvements in patients' health and a reduction in hospital admissions.[20]

In the Grampian study,[19] half of all patients (under 80) with established heart disease had at least two aspects of their medical management that were suboptimal and nearly two-thirds had at least two aspects of their health behaviour that would benefit from change. For an 'average' practice in that study this would mean:

- 30 or more individuals with heart disease taking little or no regular exercise
- a dozen smokers
- 10 obese and 30 overweight patients
- a dozen with a high-fat diet
- 30 hypertensives with suboptimal blood pressure control.

Less than a third of the patients in the study who had had a recent myo-cardial infarction were using beta-blockers, less than half with a diagnosis of heart failure were taking ACE inhibitors, and less than two-thirds were taking aspirin. Although hypertension management was good overall, with 90% of cases managed according to guidelines, lipid management was largely neglected despite the existence of local guidelines.

Hyperlipidaemia

We have discussed CHF treatment and hypertension already, but management of hyperlipidaemia in later life deserves attention because it is neglected and problematic for practitioners. Plasma lipids rise with age and the scatter of values around the mean increases, whilst older women tend to have higher cholesterol values than men, perhaps because of the early death of men with hyperlipidaemia. In the UK, a serum cholesterol of 7.0 mmoles/l is average for a woman aged 70 years.[21] Guidelines must therefore be age and gender specific to be useful in practice, and as we have seen in Chapter 3, most guidelines are not specific for age. Interpretation of lipid profiles in older women is also dif-ficult because relationships with clinical outcomes are not so apparent as they are in middle age, and falling cholesterol may signify catabolic wasting, including carcinoma of the colon. Adverse lipid profiles may occur with other diseases and clinical problems, including:

- hypothyroidism
- diabetes

- alcohol excess
- obesity
- myeloma and other immunoglobulin disorders
- chronic liver disease
- renal impairment.

The effect on lipids, and subsequently on cardiovascular risk, of optimal treatment of these conditions (where treatable) in older people is not known. However, diabetes and alcohol misuse in later life are associated with higher risk of cardiovascular disease, as is heavier weight.[22]

Treatment of primary hyperlipidaemia in patients up to 70 or 75 does reduce the incidence of, and mortality due to, cardiovascular events, including stroke,[21] especially for individuals with non-insulin dependent diabetes mellitus.[23] Treatment of hyperlipidaemia seems uncomplicated for most patients, and drug interactions in patients already taking multiple medications uncommon.[24, 25] Clinical benefits are not apparent until two years after the start of treatment, so a clinical decision needs to be made about expectation of life in each patient before treatment is initiated. The potential for benefit probably also declines with advancing age after 75, providing a rare justification for a chronological age barrier for treatment.

References

1 Gillespie N, Darbar D, Struthers AD, et al. Heart failure: a diagnostic and therapeutic dilemma in elderly patients. Age & Ageing 1998; 27(4):539–43.

2 Eccles M, Freemantle N, & Mason J North of England evidence-based development project: guidelines for angiotensin-converting enzyme inhibitors in primary care management of adults with symptomatic heart failure. British Medical Journal 1998; 316:1369–75.

3 Steeds RP & Channer KS Drug treatment in heart failure. British Medical Journal 1998; 316:567–8.

4 Davidson NC, Naas AA, Hanson JK, et al. Comparison of atrial natriuretic peptide, B-type natriuretic peptide and N terminal proatrial natriuretic peptide as indicators of left ventricular systolic dysfunction. American Journal of Cardiology 1996; 77:828–31.

5 Wallen T, Laudahl S, Hedner T, et al. Brain natriuretic peptide predicts mortality in the elderly. Heart 1997; 77:264–7.

6 Jenkinson C, Jenkinson D, Shepperd S, et al. Evaluation of treatment for congestive heart failure in patients aged 60 years and older using generic measures of health status. Age & Ageing 1997; 26:7–13.

7 O'Neill CJ, Charlett A, & Dobbs RJ Effect of captopril on functional, physiological and biochemical outcome criteria in aged heart failure patients. British Journal of Clinical Pharmacology 1992; 33:167–8.

8 The ELITE study investigators Randomised trial of losartan versus captopril in patients over 65 with heart failure. Lancet 1997; 349:747–52.

9 Ebrahim S & Davey Smith G Health promotion for cardiovascular disease among older people. Health Education Authority, London 1996.

10 Ebrahim S *Tackling diseases: towards a framework for promoting the health of older people*. Health Education Authority/Centre for Policy on Ageing, London 1996.

11 Colhoun HM, Dong W, & Poulter NR Blood pressure screening, management and control in England: results from the Health Survey for England 1994. *Journal of Hypertension* 1998; **16**:747–52.

12 Scott AK Hypertension in the elderly. *Reviews in Clinical Gerontology* 1999; **9**:39–54.

13 Breteler MMB,Claud JJ, Grobbee DE, *et al.* Cardiovascular disease and distribution of cognitive function in elderly people: the Rotterdam study. *British Medical Journal* 1994; **308**:604–8.

14 *Preventing strokes and saving lives*. The Stroke Association, London 1995.

15 Ekbom T, Lindholm LH, & Oden A A-5 year prospective, observational study of the withdrawal of antihypertensive treatment in elderly people. *Journal of International Medicine* 1994; **235**:581–8.

16 Walma EP, Hoes AW, van Dooren C, *et al.* Withdrawal of long-term diuretic medication in elderly patients: a double-blind randomised trial. *British Medical Journal* 1997; **315**:464–8.

17 Lund-Johansen P Stopping antihypertensive drug therapy in elderly people – a dangerous experiment? [editorial] *Journal of International Medicine* 1994; **235**:577–9.

18 Ebrahim S & Davey Smith G Systematic review of randomised controlled trials of multiple risk factor interventions for preventing coronary heart disease. *British Medical Journal* 1997; **314**:1666–74.

19 Campbell NC, Thain J, Deans HG, *et al.* Secondary prevention in coronary heart disease: baseline survey of provision in general practice. *British Medical Journal* 1998; **316**:1430–4.

20 Campbell NC, Thain J, Deans HG, *et al.* Secondary prevention clinics for coronary heart disease: randomised trial of effect on health. *British Medical Journal* 1998; **316**:1434–7.

21 Winder A Management of lipids in the elderly. *Journal of the Royal Society of Medicine* 1998; **91**:189–91.

22 Harris TB, Launer LJ, Madans J, *et al.* Cohort study of effect of being overweight and change in weight on risk of coronary heart diseasse in old age. *British Medical Journal* 1997; **314**:1791–4.

23 Pyorala K, Pedersen TR, Kjekshus J, *et al.* Cholesterol lowering with simvastatin improves prognosis of diabetic patients with coronary heart disease. *Diabetes Care* 1997; **20**:614–20.

24 Denke MA & Grundy SM Hypercholesterolaemia in elderly persons: resolving the treatment dilemma. *Ann. Int. Med.* 1990; **112**:780–92.

25 La Rosa JC, Applegate W, & Crouse JR Cholesterol lowering in the elderly: results of the cholesterol reduction in seniors program (CRISP) pilot study. *Arch. Intern. Med.* 1994; **154**:529–39.

CHAPTER EIGHT

Promoting continence with older adults

Mandy Wells, Continence Nurse Specialist

The health visitor had arranged a home visit to Mrs N. for an annual over-75 assessment. Mrs N. had some problems with arthritis but had not been seen by anyone at the surgery for some time. Mrs N. opened the front door to her flat, greeted the health visitor, then slowly led the way to the front room. As she did so the health visitor noticed a wet patch on the seat of her skirt. Mrs N. sat down in her armchair and the pungent scent of urine wafted across to the health visitor, seated nearby.

After settling themselves down, the health visitor started working her way through her list of areas to be explored, offering health promotion advice and suggestions as problems were identified. She then asked, 'Any problems with your bladder or bowels?'. 'No,' said Mrs N. looking the health visitor squarely in the eye. 'So, no difficulties with your waterworks?' asked the health visitor, checking the language was understood. 'No,' said Mrs N. her chin now jutting firmly forward. 'Oh dear,' thought the health visitor, and tried again. 'Sometimes as people get older they find they have to go to the toilet more often or need to get to the toilet more quickly – but you haven't experienced anything like that?' 'No,' said Mrs N. her lips tightened and pressed firmly together. The health visitor took a deep breath before starting very gently, ' I couldn't help noticing as you walked in front of me,' Mrs N.'s lips started to tremble very slightly, 'that you had a wet patch,' Mrs N.'s eyes started to glisten, 'on your skirt and a little bit of a smell of urine.' The tears started rolling silently down Mrs N.'s face. The health visitor moved forward to touch Mrs N.'s hand and give her a tissue. 'I don't mean to upset you but if you have got trouble with your waterworks, we can help. Why don't you tell me about it.' When Mrs N. could speak she told the health visitor how awful she felt. For years she had wet herself a tiny bit when she laughed too much or sneezed suddenly and she'd managed it so it wasn't a problem. Over the last year it had got a lot worse and now she really seemed to wet herself when she coughed or anything like that. She used sanitary pads to catch the urine but that wasn't working so well now.

The health visitor made a detailed assessment of all the relevant factors. She then explained it was important for the GP to give her a physical examination, for her urine to be tested to identify why this was happening and to then start appropriate treatment or action. The health visitor sat with Mrs N. while she made an appointment with the GP. The health visitor explained she would take her assessment details to the GP and also how she would use these details to order some body-worn continence pads while the investigations took place. The health visitor arranged to telephone Mrs N. after she had consulted her GP as she might have been able to help further, dependent on the GP's suggested treatment or management plan.

Introduction

GPs, nurses, and health visitors are in an excellent position to proactively address many of the risk factors associated with the onset of incontinence as well as ensure the early identification and management of continence problems. However, the combination of reticence on the part of patients and the low priority incontinence is given by health professionals creates a situation where it is ignored and badly dealt with, to the detriment of the overall well-being of the older adult and at great cost to the individual, their carers, and the state.

This chapter therefore argues for a proactive approach by the primary care team to urinary and faecal incontinence management in older people.

The prevalence of urinary incontinence

Urinary incontinence is 'a condition where involuntary loss of urine is a social or hygienic problem and is objectively demonstrable.'[1] Other definitions have been suggested which incorporate other aspects such as time periods, e.g. 'any uncontrolled urine loss in the prior 12 months without regard to severity.'[1] Numerous studies of both urinary and faecal incontinence provide a range of prevalence dependent on the definition, the research methods, and compounded by under-reporting. Urinary incontinence is not uncommon in adults, particularly women, and the incidence increases with age.[2] A review of 48 studies[3] revealed a mean prevalence in elderly women of 24.5% with a mean of 55.7% in institutionalized and impaired women. In a study specifically targeting older community-dwelling men, 29% reported uncontrolled urine leakage.[4]

Many people only report their symptoms to a health professional when they find them more worrying or can no longer cope with them. This seems particularly true for the older age group. The proportion of women aged 65 and over who delayed more than five years before discussing urinary problems with a health professional was twice that of women aged under 35 years.[5] The reluctance to consult on these problems stems from beliefs of inevitability with increased age, beliefs that nothing can be done, as well as the embarrassing nature of the problem.[6] Elderly women are thought in particular to delay consulting professionals for fear of surgery. Many elderly people use multiple strategies to prevent the sight, smell, or occurrence of urine from being detected by others.[7]

The onus is therefore on the primary care team to instigate proactive identification of individuals with continence problems – most easily through their over-75 screening programme—but to also consider how to integrate it into the care of those older people who are not part of that programme through their frequent consultation with the team for numerous other problems. Assessment tools with cue words for continence status have been shown in the USA to significantly increase the identification of urinary incontinence.[8] The case study of Mrs N. illustrates a direct case-finding approach combined with proactive questioning in the face of denial. It also illustrates the health visitor outlining her potential case management role to the older person, following consultation with the GP.

The impact of incontinence

The impact of incontinence on the emotional, social, physical and economic well-being of individuals and their carers should not be underestimated.

The experience of incontinence has a profound impact on an adult's psychological well-being. Control of bowels and bladder is fundamental to the developmental stage shift from infant to child. To lose control over the most intimate of bodily functions is experienced as humiliating and distressing at any age. Fear of this loss of control being witnessed by others leads people to curtail their social and public activities. People who are incontinent describe the psychological impact over a range of emotions, including increased levels of depression, irritability, anxiety, and feelings of hopelessness. [9] One study of women attending a urodynamic clinic found one-quarter to be as depressed, anxious, and phobic as psychiatric patients.[10] Increased levels of social isolation are one significant impact[11] which may compound the psychological impact. Chapter 9 considers the underdetection and treatment of depression in the elderly and should be considered when supporting patients with continence problems. A number of recent studies have described the negative impact of incontinence on sexuality and sexual relationships.[12] They have almost always looked at women's experience and exclusively at women under 60.[13] Quality of life issues are important, therefore more than just the mechanics of urinating needs to be addressed in treating and managing incontinence.

People with incontinence tend to stick near to home and feel uncomfortable about travelling too far or using public transport. This factor has been exacerbated by the decrease in the number of public lavatories that has occurred over the past decades. Lack or ease of access to lavatories in GP surgeries may be significant for some people in their decision to consult the GP.

Living with a person who is incontinent can be distressing as well as physically exhausting. Coping with a dementing loved one who urinates in the corners of their shared home or smears faeces across clothes and furniture, puts extraordinary levels of stress on carers. In these circumstances, treatment options may be limited but strategies for management essential. Studies in America have shown not only that incontinence has been a significant factor in the decision by carers to place their demented relative in a nursing home, but one study has demonstrated it to be a predictor of institutionalization.[14]

The economic impact for the individual and family is hard to assess. Prior to consultation with a health professional, people purchase incontinence management products – often in the form of sanitary protection.[15] They may also use old towels and bed linen as their primary protection , with the consequent frequent laundry costs.[16] Purchase of these items and the additional laundry can represent a significant expense[17, 18] to someone who is already struggling to exist on state pensions, reducing the money available for other essentials such as food and warmth.

In 1991 the Department of Health estimated the NHS spent 50 million pounds directly on pads and appliances, and a further £18 million was spent through prescriptions for appliances.[19] Incontinence management products are the financial responsibility of the health service to provide. This is usually managed through a community trust for community-living adults. Each area will have its own assessment, ordering, and delivery system with weekly limits on supplies. Access to incontinence laundry services comes within the domain of the local authorities and is subject to local eligibility criteria and charging systems. There has been a paucity of work directed at calculating the total cost of incontinence, both direct and indirect. Further work needs to be developed into calculating the costs of incontinence for older adults. It is an issue that PCGs will look to address within both their clinical governance agenda but also within their prescribing budget.

Aetiology of urinary incontinence in the elderly

The aetiology of urinary incontinence in the elderly is complex, demonstrating the interplay between associated factors,[20] which are outlined in Box 8.1.

Box 8.1 *Risk factors associated with urinary incontinence*

- Immobility/chronic degenerative disease
- Congestive heart failure
- Diabetes
- Concurrent medication
- Impaired cognition
- Smoking
- Environmental barriers
- Faecal impaction
- Obesity
- Neurological disease/injury
- Parity
- Oestrogen depletion
- Urinary tract infection

Multiple and interacting factors contribute to the development of urinary incontinence, especially in the frail older person.[21] Identification and management of problems, such as inability to undo clothing in time at the toilet, need as much attention as the diagnosis of underlying pathology and point to the need for systematic assessment of all potential factors.

The assessment of incontinence

We advocate a systematic approach agreed across a primary care team, preferably using a single assessment protocol based on expert consensus guidelines[22,23] and customized to the particular area. The following outlines the key aspects of the assessment which are concerned with:

- differential diagnosis
- identification and management of reversible conditions that cause or contribute to urinary incontinence
- quality of life for the person and their carers
- management and containment of the incontinence.

(1) **The presenting symptoms and history of incontinence** – a detailed exploration of the symptoms is important as is clarifying the most bothersome symptoms to the older person. This may be especially important in decisions regarding treatment and management. Box 8.2 provides a reminder of the classification of urinary incontinence with its associated symptoms.

(2) **Impact on the person's quality of life** – for example reducing social contact outside the home, impact on sexuality, evidence of depression.

(3) **Past medical history** – for example onset following childbirth, stroke, pelvic surgery.

(4) **Associated disease** – for example dementia, diabetes, neurological disease, spinal cord disease.

(5) **Disability and impairment** – for example resulting from arthritis, parkinsonism.

(6) **Environmental difficulties** – for example the toilet is too low, far away, or via stairs.

(7) **Current medications and drug use** – for example diuretics, sedatives, anti-parkinsonian, alcohol consumption, smoking.

(8) **Dietary intake and fluids.**

Physical and other investigations

(1) **Urinalysis** to detect conditions that are associated with, or contribute to, urinary incontinence, such as haematuria (suggestive of infection, stone, or cancer) and glucosuria (which may cause polyuria and contribute to symptoms). Dipstick methods are available to detect bacteriuria. Although there is a clear relationship between symptomatic urinary tract infection (UTI) (dysuria) and incontinence, the relationship between asymptomatic bacteriuria and incontinence remains controversial.[28] Although there is some debate about the treatment of asymptomatic bacteriuria, it would appear appropriate to treat the bacteriuria and observe the effect on incontinence symptoms. This is particularly pertinent if the bacteriuria has not been previously evaluated or treated.

(2) **Physical examination** is an imperative. Unfortunately a number of

Box 8.2 *Types of urinary incontinence*[24]

Detrusor instability: urge incontinence

Urge incontinence is usually, but not always, associated with the uro-dynamic finding of involuntary detrusor contractions, referred to as detrusor instability. This is associated with urgency to void, frequency, voiding with little or no warning, and nocturia.[25] It is the most common cause of urinary incontinence in the elderly.[26]

Stress incontinence

Stress urinary incontinence is defined as urine loss coincident with an increase in intra-abdominal pressure, in the absence of a detrusor contraction or an overdistended bladder. Clinically it presents as the voluntary loss of urine on coughing, sneezing, laughing, or performing other physical activities. This is present in about 85% of women presenting with incontinence.[27] It is usually associated with bladder outlet incompetence through weakness of the supporting pelvic floor muscles.

Mixed incontinence

It is not uncommon for people to complain of both urge and stress symptoms. This is termed mixed urinary incontinence. This is particularly common in post-menopausal women. The most important aspect of this type of incontinence is identifying which is the most 'bothersome' symptom for the individual. This is the symptom that should then be targeted.

Overflow incontinence

This term is used to describe the involuntary loss of urine associated with overdistension of the bladder. It can be caused by a number of different conditions. These include bladder outlet or urethral obstruction which is most commonly seen in men with prostatic hyperplasia. This type of incontinence is less common in women. However, it may occur as a complication of surgical intervention of an anti-incontinence operation or because of severe pelvic organ prolapse.

An underactive or acontractile detrusor muscle can also lead to overdistension and overflow. The causes of this are numerous, including neurological disorders such as strokes or multiple sclerosis, diabetes, and medication side-effects. In some individuals this can also be idiopathic.

studies show that in the primary health care setting patients are rarely examined.[29] *Abdominal palpation* to detect masses which can relate to a full bladder or constipation. *Pelvic examination* to detect genital atrophy, pelvic organ prolapse, pelvic mass, and paravaginal muscle tone. *Rectal examination* is essential to rule out constipation or impaction. In addition, in men with suspected outlet obstruction, a rectal examination is essential. A general examination for neurological abnormalities is also indicated.

3. **A post-void residual volume** is an essential component of the assessment of urinary incontinence.[30] This can be estimated using abdominal palpation and percussion, or by urethral catheterization, or by using portable ultrasound equipment (the latter being available from most continence services). In clinical practice it is generally accepted that a residual volume below 100 ml is normal.

4. **Detailed description of the pattern of frequency, volume of voiding, and fluid intake obtained through a week-long frequency–volume chart.** Charting, as shown in Figure 8.1, will provide more objective information on the number of incontinent episodes, the frequency of micturition (diurnal and nocturnal), and functional bladder capacity. These type of charts can be used to inform treatment decisions as well as monitoring progress.

This type of assessment list lends itself to protocol agreement between primary care professionals to ensure all aspects are covered – some being undertaken by the GP, some by the health visitor, district nurse, or practice nurse.

Referral for more specialist evaluation should be considered against the following criteria although of course this is not prescriptive in every situation – not least because it may not be desired by the patient:

- uncertain diagnosis
- difficulties in developing an appropriate treatment plan
- failure to respond to the treatment/management plan after an appropriate period
- the presence of other complicating morbidity.

Figure 8.1 Example of a frequency–volume chart.

Time	Day 1				
	Urinated in toilet	Small amount of incontinence	Large amount of incontinence	Reason for incontinence	Drinks/ liquid taken
e.g. 6 a.m. 7 a.m.	✓	✓		sneezed	*cup of tea*
Number of pads used today =	*Any other comments*				

There appears to be no consensus, however, on the requirement for all patients to undergo urodynamic testing in order for a diagnosis to be made.[31] Within the clinical governance agenda of PCGs this may be an area that needs local consensus criteria in order to ensure equity of provision for all older people with continence problems.

Treatment of urinary incontinence

The primary aim of the treatment and support of incontinence in older people has to be the avoidance of social isolation.[32] Studies have shown that treatment provided within the general practice setting can lead to improved continence status.[33] However, this is not always the experience of patients. One study[34] which tracked people with overactive bladder problems found that 75% of continence sufferers who discussed their problems with a health care professional said that the doctor/nurse to whom they were referred understood their concern, but 36% suggested a 'wait and see' policy, 27% said their condition was not serious enough at present, and 26% said that it was something one had to live with.

There is evidence that primary care professionals perceive themselves as needing more education in this area before becoming more proactive in the prevention and management of incontinence. In one survey, GPs were asked how they had received training in continence care[35] sixty-two per cent had received continence care training as part of their general medicine training, while only 34% had attended further postgraduate courses. Only 9% of doctors had received specialist training in continence care. Two per cent responded that they had received their training from district nurses, whilst 14% had received no training at all. When asked about the adequacy of training, 43% believed it to be inadequate. This is clearly an issue for PCGs in looking at education and training provision within their clinical governance brief.

The evidence base for continence treatment and management is lacking in many aspects. A number of consensus guidelines have been produced[36,37] to assist clinicians in their decision-making when assessing and treating urinary incontinence. The treatment categories are:

* behavioural
* pharmacological
* surgical.

The primary care options are outlined below and summarized in the Brief Guide to Urinary Incontinence in Adults, developed by the Continence Foundation[38] and reproduced in Table 8.1.

Management of stress incontinence: pelvic floor re-education

Stress incontinence is usually treated conservatively through teaching pelvic floor exercises.[39] Unfortunately, like so much of continence management,

Table 8.1 *A brief guide to bladder control problems in adults*

Minimum history	Minimum examination	Minimum investigation	Referral options
• when started • frequency, amount of leakage • current management, fluid intake • effect on lifestyle	• abdomen • PR, PV • relevant neurological assessment	• frequency/volume chart • residual urine estimation (scan or in/out catheterizaton) • dipstick/MSSU	

Causes and symptoms	Possible underlying problems	Treatment	Minimum investigation	Referral options
Stress incontinence: leaking with coughing, laughing, exercise	Urethral sphincter incompetence, pelvic floor weakness	Pelvic floor therapy, urethral appliances, surgical intervention		Continence specialist nurse, physiotherapist, urogynaecologist, urologist
Voiding inefficiency: continual dribbling, weak flow, hesitancy, incomplete emptying, intermittent stream, straining to void	Bladder outlet obstruction (prostatic enlargement, urethral stricture, faecal impaction)	Clear any impaction; otherwise, surgical referral required		Prostate assessment clinic, urologist
	Detrusor failure (secondary to neurological disease)	Clean intermittent catheterizaton if post-micturition residual >150 ml		Continence specialist nurse, specialist continence service
Detrusor overactivity: urinary urgency, frequency (>8/24h), urge incontinence, latchkey morning urgency	Idiopathic detrusor overactivity	Check residual volume, advice on fluid intake, bladder retraining programme anticholinergic drugs		Continence specialist nurse, specialist continence service

				*other referrals
	Detrusor overactivity secondary to neurological disease (e.g. MS)		Urologist, urogynaecologist, incontinence specialist nurse	
	Cystitis, classical (internal) dysuria secondary to UTI	Appropriate antibiotic therapy. Refer if recurrent		
	Atrophic urethritis or vaginitis, external dysuria	Topical oestrogen replacement or systematic HRT	Gynaecologist, specialist continence service	
	Bladder calculus	Surgical referral	Urologist	
Cognitive impairment	CNS disease (dementia, delirium)	Exclude iatrogenic causes; appropriate toileting programmes; minimize handicap	Community nurse, community psychiatric nurse, specialist continence service	
Physical impairment	Impaired dexterity/mobility		Physiotherapist, occupational therapist	
Enuresis: bed wetting	Detrusor instability, prostatism, immobility, primary nocturnal enuresis	As for underlying condition. Antidiuretic in some cases	Specialist continence service	
Possible confounding factors: anticholinergics, diuretics, alph-adrenoreceptor blockers, calcium channel blockers, sedatives	Review environment, e.g. ease of access to WC	**Containment during investigation or if problem regarded as intractable:** • body worn and bed pads • timed voiding programmes • in-dwelling catheter (last resort)	• urethral appliances • sheaths and urinals	geriatrician/ physician

there is a paucity of robust evidence concerning pelvic floor exercises. A number of studies investigating the value of this technique with older women have consistently found an improvement in the level of stress incontinence following a programme of pelvic floor exercises.[40] The one randomized controlled trial conducted on older women found that they will accept and maintain a regime of pelvic floor exercises and that beneficial effects are maintained at least six months after completion of the initial intervention.[41] The form the pelvic floor re-education should take has also been debated.[42] A RCT of three treatment interventions versus no treatment was undertaken in women aged 24–50.[43] The interventions included pelvic floor exercises (8–12 contractions three times a day and exercise in groups with skilled physical therapists once a week), or electrical stimulation or vaginal cones. The improvement in muscle strength was significantly greater after pelvic floor exercises than in any of the other groups. The efficacy of vaginal cones is much debated and the research evidence on their effectiveness is limited. They may help however to increase the strength of the muscle contraction and provide proprioceptive feedback, and are considered a low-risk therapy for stress incontinence.[44] However, it has been shown that many women find them difficult to use.[45] Other techniques such as biofeedback and electrical stimulation are of value,[46] but are in the main used by specialist physiotherapists and continence nurses. In considering the possibility of referring an older person for surgical opinion, the most important issue to be taken into consideration is whether the operation will improve the quality of life of the patient.[47]

Management of stress incontinence: urethral and vaginal appliances

Over the past several years there have been a variety of urethral or vaginal appliances manufactured. These are generally occlusive devices which are intended to eliminate or reduce leakage. However, the efficacy of the use of urethral appliances and in addition vaginal appliances is debatable. Appliances tend to come on the market and then disappear without trace. Continence nurse specialists and specialist physiotherapists keep up to date on availability. If a patient is greatly concerned with the level of their incontinence and enquires about an appliance, they should consequently be referred to these practitioners.

Voiding inefficiency

The key elements here when a patient presents with symptoms of voiding inefficiency are to exclude faecal impaction and, in men, prostate enlargement. Physical examination is therefore imperative. If faecal impaction is present this needs to be treated and the patient then reassessed. On indication of prostate enlargement, the patient should be referred to a urologist and prostate assessment clinic for an in-depth assessment.

Voiding inefficiency due to detrusor failure with a post-micturition residual urine above 150 ml responds well to a programme of *clean intermittent catheterization*. This is a procedure that has been found to be effective in managing voiding inefficiently problems for many years.[48,49] It is usually carried out every three to six hours. In the elderly, however, as the fluid output tends to be lower, a less frequent regime of twice-daily catheterization may prove adequate.[50] It can be performed by either patients themselves or their caregivers, using clean catheters. Patients need to be motivated and have good manual dexterity, again pointing to the importance of the initial assessment process. In addition they need to be taught by a confident and experienced health care professional. For many older people this procedure may have to be performed by community nursing staff.

Some patients may have concurrent detrusor overactivity in conjunction with voiding inefficiently. It is important that a regime of intermittent catheterization is commenced in addition to any other treatment regime.

Detrusor overactivity: education and bladder retraining

A programme of non-pharmaceutical treatment is the first option to treat detrusor overactivity. This is particularly true for older patients who are more likely to experience side-effects of a medication due to co-morbidity and changes in pharmacokinetics.[51] Again associated voiding inefficiency should be excluded through investigation for residual urine.

People with urgency and urge incontinence tend to reduced their fluid intake in order to reduce the severity of the symptoms.[52] These patients need to be re-educated on the importance of drinking approximately 1.5–2 litres of fluid a day. In addition patients need to be made aware of the diuretic effect of constituents in everyday drinks such as caffeine and alcohol, one study having shown that caffeine abstinence helped to significantly reduce the incidence of urinary incontinence among psychogeriatric patients.[53] A North American study identified that 60% of caffeine was consumed in coffee, 16% in soft drinks, and less than 2% in chocolate.[54] It can be argued that in the United Kingdom a large amount of caffeine could be consumed in tea. When restricting caffeine it must be noted that patients can get withdrawal symptoms. Headache is the most common symptom with fatigue, anxiety, and irritability also occurring. These withdrawal symptoms usually occur 12–24 hours after the last intake of caffeine, peak at 20–48 hours, and take up to a week to resolve.[55]

Bladder retraining

Bladder retraining means the patient learns to resist the desire to void, thus stretching the bladder and reducing its activity. The actual mechanism behind the success of bladder retraining has been debated.[56] It could be mechanical in that by stretching the bladder you can dampen down the effect of the unstable. In contrast some argue it could be psychological in that patients learn not to go 'just in case' and how to develop better bladder habits. This treatment has been found to work on its own in the absence of medications.[57] It has been used successfully in a geriatric out-patient department where an 80% reduction in incontinence episodes was noted.[58] The primary care studies that have used bladder retraining in their care packages have demonstrated improvement in continence status.[59] However, patients do need to be motivated and encouraged to perform the technique as it can be uncomfortable and in the short term could increase the number of incontinence episodes. The importance of a case management approach is vital in sustaining the patient through the process.

A retraining programme gradually increases the time between voiding, aiming from three to four hours.[60] There are two main types of programmes taught, although there is no evidence of greater efficacy. The first encourages the person to resist the desire to void as long as they possibly can with the aim of getting the frequency of voids down to six a day. The second has the same aim but instructs the patient to gradually extend the length of time they wait before they go to pass urine once they have felt the urge. Both methods use a bladder chart or urinary diary. These provide a permanent record for baseline and subsequent evaluation of symptoms.[61] They are useful to patients in that they provide a feedback of improvement in their frequency and in their incontinent episodes, aiding motivation.

Medication in the treatment of incontinence

Anticholinergic drugs

At the time of writing this chapter there are four drugs in general use for the treatment of detrusor overactivity. The use of drugs in the elderly requires special consideration. Decreased renal clearance is primarily responsible for increased sensitivity, but reduced organ reserve, loss of carrier proteins, and the increased fat–water ratio also contribute.[62]

Oxybutynin hydrochloride

Oxybutynin is a tertiary amine and a muscarinic antagonist with potent antispasmodic activity. The recommended dosage is 5 mg three times a day,[63] however it is advisable to start on a lower dose of 2.5 mg twice a day as its side-effects can often lead to poor patient compliance. The side-effects involve a dry mouth, constipation, reflux oesophagitis (the usual reason for withdrawal of the medication), dry skin, blurred vision, constipation, nausea, abdominal discomfort, facial flushing, some minor ankle swelling, and difficulty with micturition.[64] There have been reported interactions between oxybutynin and phenothizines, levodopa, digoxin, and tricyclic antidepressants. Care must therefore be taken if concurrent treatment takes place.[65] Contraindications include intestinal obstruction, severe ulcerative colitis, bladder outlet obstruction, glaucoma, or myasthenia gravis. In older people caution should be exercised in the presence of hepatic or renal impairment, severe cardiac disease, and autonomic neuropathy. Special care should be taken with hiatus hernia, especially in the elderly if associated with reflux oesophagitis.

Tolterodine

Tolterodine is a newer, muscarinic receptor antagonist. It shows selectivity for the bladder rather than salivary glands.[56] It has been found to be as efficacious as oxybutynin at a dose of 5 mg three times a day, but without the severity of side-effects – particularly dry mouth.[67]

Propiverine hydrochloride

Propiverine hydrochloride is another newer drug whose mode of action involves both antimuscarinic and calcium-channel blocking properties.[68] This drug has recently been introduced onto the UK market. It appears to be as efficacious as oxybutynin but once again with fewer side-effects. Its half-life allows administration of a twice-daily dose (15mg), but this can be increased to three times daily with an increase in response.[69]

Flavoxate hydrochloride

Flavoxate hydrochloride is a drug with papverine-like properties. Although this drug is still routinely used, from the data available it is difficult to reach a conclusion about its value over a placebo.[70] However, it is associated with fewer side-effects than other medications, the main complaints being of nausea and vomiting.

Oestrogen

The role of oestrogen replacement therapy in the treatment of urinary incontinence remains unclear with few controlled studies reported.[71] Knowledge regarding the effect of the medication are incomplete despite widespread anecdotal evidence. Its use in primary care is therefore debatable. One instance where it might be considered useful is in the management of recurrent urinary infection.[72] Oestrogen withdrawal is associated with a fall in the levels of intravaginal glycogen on which lactobacilli depend. These bacteria cease to colonize the vagina, which is then occupied by colonic organisms. The atrophy of the urethelium encourages colonization by gram-negative faecal organisms and the urethelium becomes more adherent for these bacteria. Oestrogen replacement therapy may reverse this process and give protection to elderly women with recurrent UTIs.[73]

Table 8.1 from the Continence Foundation[74] summarizes proactive care of urinary incontinence. Studies show that there is a high level of satisfaction with incontinence treatment managed from within primary care.[75] We would argue that more primary care teams could become more proactive in the management of these problems. In particular, nurses have the potential to become more active in those options which involve patient education and case management.

> Mr D. was a 68 year old catholic priest, formerly an army officer – and wet the bed at night all his life. Mr D. hid his problem using a variety of strategies. During his 25 years in the Army, Mr D. achieved all his ambitions, despite the enuresis. But during all those years he never sought medical advice for his problem for fear that he would be thrown out of the Services.

It was only when Mr D. retired from the Army and became a parish priest that he first approached a GP with his problem. The GP immediately referred him to a consultant urologist who carried out a series of tests to check his bladder and bowels were functioning properly. There was nothing obviously wrong that could be corrected through surgery so, over the next few years, the urologist prescribed a range of medications including an anti-diuretic hormone to restrict the output of the kidneys at night. Unfortunately, unlike a lot of people with enuresis, Mr D.'s problem persisted. 'I think if I had asked for help when I was younger – before the bedwetting became such an ingrained habit – it's quite possible they would have been able to cure me'. Nevertheless, he is glad that he did eventually seek treatment. 'It's true that they haven't managed to cure me but the continence advisors and district nurses I have been put in touch with have helped me enormously by teaching me how to manage my incontinence. If I want, I can get a condom and bag system on prescription to wear at night to collect the urine. And through the district nurse I get a regular supply of absorbent pads delivered to my house every month. They've also given me a waterproof mattress cover.'

Mr D. clearly felt great relief in being able to discuss the problem and find assistance in containing the consequences 'For so many years I kept it secret and it was a terrible burden. I feel so much happier now that I talk about it openly. I'm no longer ashamed and I don't see why anyone else with incontinence should be.'

We will return to the wider issues in the management of continence once we have considered faecal incontinence.

Prevalence of bowel continence problems

The impact of faecal incontinence mirrors and amplifies those described for urinary incontinence. It is clear that underestimates of prevalence are common because of reluctance to admit to this symptom. It has even been described as a 'subject too distasteful to mention.'[76] It is indeed still firmly hidden by the patient.[77]

Prevalence studies show faecal incontinence in the community as more common than health care professionals previously realized especially in the female population – often the result of damage to the anal sphincters in childbirth.[78] A community-based prevalence study in the USA cites 2.2% of the respondents reporting anal incontinence.[79] Of these, 30% were over 65 years of age and 63% were female. In the UK, a study by the MRC Incontinence Study Team[80] of 15,904 adults over the age of 40 found 8% of those aged 65–84 and 16% of those aged over 85 reporting faecal incontinence. However, double incontinence was also found to be common. This group defined faecal incontinence as leakage from bowels several times a month, irrespective of volume. They highlighted that a consensus on definitions of faecal incontinence is needed to avoid inconstancies in epidemiological studies and to aid treatment in the primary care setting.

The most common cause of faecal incontinence in older adults is believed to be constipation.[81] Recent studies of the prevalence of constipation in adults in the UK demonstrate 20% of people over the age of 65 being affected.[82] The common definition of constipation is defecation less frequently than every third day.[83] However, there are people who believe daily defecation is normal and important for maintenance of health – any other pattern for them represents constipation. Others believe they are constipated in that they have to strain to defecate.[84] The actual diagnosis of constipation should be based on the 'Rome' diagnostic criteria devised by a working group on bowel disease:[85]

(1) straining at defecation for at least a quarter of the time
(2) lumpy and/or hard stools for at least a quarter of the time
(3) a sensation of incomplete evacuation for at least a quarter of the time
(4) two or fewer bowel movements per week.

Constipation interferes with daily living and impairs well-being.[86] Approximately 6% of a frail, community-living, elderly population counted constipation as one of their top three health concerns.[87]

Assessment and treatment of bowel incontinence

The key elements of an assessment reflect those of urinary continence assessment. A detailed understanding of types of stool and frequency of problems is aided by pictorial stool charts (usually available through specialist continence nurses and some continence products manufacturers) and bowel habit diaries (Figure 8.2).

A stepwise progression in dealing with constipation is advocated by many commentators and supported in the systematic review of the effectiveness of laxatives in older adults.[88] It concludes there is no evidence to indicate efficacy of one laxative over another – such as the more expensive stimulant laxatives – and suggests that the cheapest should therefore be used. There is little robust

Figure 8.2 Example of diet and bowel diary.

Day and time (please write this diary for 7 days)	Please note down food and drink taken	Bowel action with information about the type of stool/wind/straining
e.g. *Monday* *7 a.m.* *8 a.m.*	*cup of hot water* *cup of tea and two pieces of white toast with butter and marmalade*	*sat on the toilet–just wind and tummy pains*

evidence on best prevention and management options and guidance tends to develop from expert consensus. Figure 8.3 provides an overview.

The prevention of constipation and faecal impaction is a key aim. Faecal incontinence can be due to faecal impaction. When a patient is impacted, a watery or mushy stool seeps around the obstructing faecal mass. In this instance the initial aim of the treatment is to empty the rectum and colon by combined enemas, rectal washouts, and aperients. Prevention and management of chronic constipation then becomes the aim.

The treatment options for faecal incontinence remain fairly limited and under-researched. They include bowel habit training and drug therapy for liquid stools once the cause has been established.

Bowel training is the first-line, non-invasive treatment choice. This includes:

- a regular schedule for sitting on the toilet in line with the individual's previous habits
- a fluid intake of a minimum of eight cups/glasses of fluid a day
- a diet including a minimum of five portions of fruit and vegetables a day (excluding potatoes) and adequate other dietary fibre
- as much exercise as possible within the constraints of the individual's ability.

Figure 8.3 *Guidance on assessment and management of constipation.*

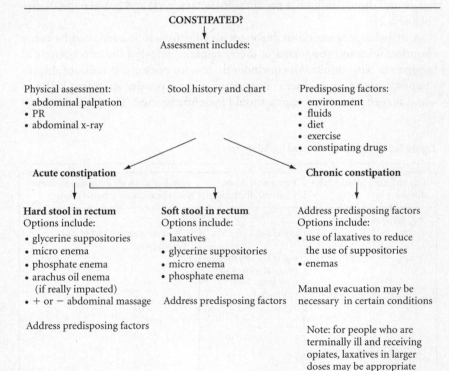

CONSTIPATED?

Assessment includes:

Physical assessment:
- abdominal palpation
- PR
- abdominal x-ray

Stool history and chart

Predisposing factors:
- environment
- fluids
- diet
- exercise
- constipating drugs

Acute constipation

Chronic constipation

Hard stool in rectum
Options include:
- glycerine suppositories
- micro enema
- phosphate enema
- arachus oil enema (if really impacted)
- + or − abdominal massage

Address predisposing factors

Soft stool in rectum
Options include:
- laxatives
- glycerine suppositories
- micro enema
- phosphate enema

Address predisposing factors

Address predisposing factors
Options include:
- use of laxatives to reduce the use of suppositories
- enemas

Manual evacuation may be necessary in certain conditions

Note: for people who are terminally ill and receiving opiates, laxatives in larger doses may be appropriate

Loperamide and codeine phosphate help deal with incontinence by making the stool firmer. There is also some evidence that loperamide also directly reduces the sensation of urgency and increases resting anal sphincter tone.[89] Both drugs can be individually titrated to reach their maximum effect. For some patients in whom passive leakage is a major problem, they can stop spontaneous evacuation by using these drugs to constipate themselves. Artificial means such as suppositories or enemas can then be used to empty the bowel at a planned and convenient time.[90,91]

Bowel problem management is summarized in the Continence Foundation guide, reproduced in Table 8.2.

Management of continence problems

Alongside the treatment options – and in some instances instead of – older people and their carers need advice and help on the associated management of the problem. Continence specialist nurses can provide expert help and advice to primary care professionals in formulating these as well as treatment plans.

Containment is one of the most important issues to a person who has continence problems. Continence products include continence pads with pants (reusable and disposable). The same types of pads can be used for the containment of urine and faeces. These are funded through health authority budgets and usually provided by community health services. Urological products (catheters, drainage bags, sheaths) are prescription-only items and are included in the new *Nurse Prescribers' Formulary*.[92] A faecal collection pouch has been available for use on prescription, since 1986. This has been used successfully with very acutely ill, terminally ill, and bed-bound patients, where it can improve dignity and reduce the distress and pain caused by frequent perineal cleansing.

Associated advice and education is important for the person with incontinence. The more cognitively or physically impaired the patient the more carers, family members, and formal paid carers will need the advice and teaching. This includes discussion of:

- appropriate fluid levels and diet – including fibre intake (this may need more detailed exploration to identify and eliminate foods which create excess of foul-smelling flatus for that person)
- aids – containment products and their use
- skin care in order to prevent excoriation and in less mobile people the creation of pressure sores, including frequent washing and the use of barrier creams
- the correct disposal of clinical waste under the local arrangements between the local authority and health authority
- the importance of laundering soiled clothes in hot, soapy water to remove the residue and prevent offensive smells as well as criteria for access to local authority incontinence laundry services
- the use of plastic covers in beds and chairs to prevent spoiling these items and their becoming a source of offensive odour

Table 8.2 *A brief guide to bowel control problems in adults*

Impairment	Minimum history	Possible causes	Usual symptoms	Minimum examination	Treatment	Possible referrals
Anal sphincter weakness or damage	• nature (urge or passive) • when started/how often now • nature of stool/evacuation difficulties/rectal bleeding • effect on lifestyle • past medical, surgical, obstetric, and drug history	Childbirth Anal surgery Direct trauma Rectal prolapse Idiopathic weakness	Urgency/urge incontinence (external anal sphincter) Passive soiling (internal anal sphincter)	• abdomen • PR • proctoscopy/sigmoidoscopy if indicated	Sphincter exercises if weak Surgical repair if simple disruption Induce firm stool with diet or medication (no clear surgical options)	Colorectal surgeon Gastroenterologist Geriatrician District nurse Neurologist Continence specialist nurse Physiotherapist

Intestinal hurry	Infection Inflammatory bowel disease Irritable bowel syndrome Drug-induced	Frequency, urgency, urge incontinence, loose stool	Treat underlying cause Constipating agents
Impaction with overflow	Immobility Physical or mental frailty Medication Dementia	Passive loss of 'spurious diarrhoea' or of solid stool	Disimpact, then keep rectum empty
Neurological disease or damage	Spinal injury Multiple sclerosis	Reflex incontinence or impaction with overflow	Regulate bowel habit Control evacuation with laxatives, evacuants, or irrigation

urgent referral: recent change of bowel habit; rectal bleeding; pain. Referral for anorectal physiology studies and anal ultrasound if conservative measures failing within 1–2 months.

Table 8.3

Suggested outcome indicator	Rationale
Reduction in the delay of presentation with urinary incontinence	Early treatment for urinary incontinence should reduce the time spent suffering distress, and patients should feel able to approach and elicit such help from their doctor or other relevant health clinicians. This indicator, by identifying changes in the numbers who delay seeking help or the scale of that delay, will reflect to some extent the success of local campaigns which aim to reduce the stigma attached to the condition and increase the awareness and use of local services.
Clinical assessment rates following presentation with urinary incontinence in a GP population	Studies of people with incontinence have revealed that although more people are now consulting their GPs about incontinence than previously, the actions carried out by GPs still appear to be suboptimal and show considerable geographic variation. This indicator will measure the number of patients whose initial presentation with incontinence led to follow-up actions (1. abdominal and vaginal or rectal examination; 2. urine specimen taken) occuring within 30 days of the initial presentation. Having undertaken these appropriate follow-up actions suggests that a good history has been taken. This indicator will reflect, to some extent, the failure to assess appropriately.
Rate of referral following presentation with urinary incontinence in a GP population	This indicator's aim is to void or reduce the adverse effects of incontinence that can be caused by delayed diagnosis and treatment. It aims to measure the number of patients whose initial presentation with incontinence was followed by a referral to a relevant continence specialist – either medical, nursing, or therapy. The indicator will measure the referral pattern one month after presentation, divided by the number of initial presentations.

- the use of appropriate cleaning materials to clean urine and faeces from floors, walls, and household items–eliminating odour problems and minimizing risks of cross infection
- advice on hand-washing and precautions for infection control both for the individual and any other carers
- advice on odour management, particularly of faeces.

The provision of aids (such as urinals and commodes), pads, and pants is organized differently across the UK, an issue for consideration in national service frameworks if not PCGs. It is clear that the economic impact of managing continence has led to disparate availability of continence products to older people[93] through the NHS. Invariably there will be a catalogue of products, with costs and quantities, provided to the health professionals – usually nurses – who take responsibility for the assessment, ordering, and review processes. In some areas aids and home adaptations will only be available through assessment by the local authority occupational therapist. The important issue is that the primary care professional is fully cognisant of the local systems and utilizes them to full benefit for the older person.

Clinical effectiveness and continence

While the drive is for evidence-based clinical care in continence care, there remains a lack of vigorous, robust scientific evidence into which conservative treatments work – an indication perhaps of the low status the condition has. The one exception to this is in the field of medications where good evidence is available on which drugs are effective in the treatment of different forms of incontinence. The guidance therefore tends to be based on expert consensus for best practice. The Eli Lilly National Clinical Audit Centre has produced an audit tool[94] as has the Royal College of Physcians[95] which provides a useful way into examining areas for improvement in clinical practice and service delivery. In addition the Department of Health has developed evidence-based outcome indicators for use in all areas of health care delivery and by all professional groups.[96] It will be interesting to see how many PCGs use these in their clinical governance work. The aim of health indicators is that they should be relevant; reliable; responsive, and research based – pointing out issues for further improvement. Several indicators which relate to care in the community and in general practice have been stated by the outcome indicator working party and are given in Table 8.3.

PCGs will need to consider the use of some of these tools and indicators in considering continence care of old people within its clinical governance framework, particularly in highlighting the issues for local training and education strategies. This may increasingly come to the fore as nurse prescribing becomes more widespread – aperients and urological products feature heavily in the *Nurse Prescribers Formulary*.

Conclusion

Incontinence can have a major impact on an individual's life. There is a growing body of evidence that there are effective conservative treatments for urine incontinence suitable to be undertaken within primary care. Primary care groups, primary care teams, and individual community practitioners are in an excellent position to be able to change the culture of incontinence care. The introduction of nurse prescribing will provide a springboard to a more proactive approach to continence case management in primary care, placing it firmly on the PCG clinical governance agenda.

References

1 Abrahams P, Blaiva JG, Stanton S L, *et al.* Standardisation of terminology of lower urinary tract function. *Neurol.Urondyn.* 1988; **7**:403–27.

2 Pharmacia & Upjohn (1997) *The Multinational Tracking Survey: overactive bladder symptoms.* Sifo Research and Consulting AB.

3 Thuroff JW, Chartier-Kastler E, Corcus J, *et al.* Medical treatment and medical side-effects in urinary incontinence in the elderly. *World Journal of Urology* 1998; **16**:S48–S61.

4 Umlauf M G & Sherman S Symptoms of urinary incontinence among older community-dwelling men. J.W.O.C.N. 1996; **23**(6):314–21.

5 Norton P A, MacDonald L D, Sedgwick PM, *et al.* Distress and delay associated with urinary incontinence, frequency, and urgency in women. *British Medical Journal,* 1988; **297**:1187–9.

6 Harrison GL & Memel DS Urinary incontinence in women: its prevalence and management in a health promotion clinic. *British Journal of General Practice* 1994; **44**(381): 149–52.

7 Talbot L A & Cos M Differences in coping strategies among community-residing older adults with functional urinary continence, dysfunctional urinary continence and actual urinary incontinence. *Ostomy/Wound Management* 1995; **41**(10):30–7..

8 USA Agency for Health Care Policy and Research (1996) *Urinary incontinence clinical guidelines.* found at http://text.nlm.nih.gov/tempfiles/is/tempD164316

9 P Norton, *et al.* op cit.

10 Maccauley AJ , Stern RS, & Stanton SL Psychological aspects of 211 female patients attending a urodynamic unit. *Journal of Psychosomatic Research* 1991; **35**(1):1–10.

11 Grimby A,Milsom I , Molander U, *et al.* The influence of urinary incontinence on the quality of life of elderly women. Age and Ageing 1993; **22**(2):82–9.

12 Kelleher C J, Cardozo L D, Wise DBG *et al.*, The impact of urinary incontinence on sexual function. *Neurological Urodynamics*, 1992; **11**(4):359–60.

13 Hilton P , Urinary incontinence during sexual intercourse: a common but rarely volunteered symptom. *British Journal of Obstetrics and Gynaecology,* 1988; **95**(4):377–81.

14 O'Donnell BF, Drachman DA, *et al.* Incontinence and troublesome behaviours predict institutionalisation in dementia. *Journal of Geriatric Psychiatry and Neurology* 1992; **5**:42–52.

15 O'Brien J, Austin M , Sethis P , *et al.* Urinary incontinence: prevalence, need for treatment, and effectiveness of intervention by nurse. *British Medical Journal* 1991; **303**(6813):1308–12.

16 Dowell C J, Bryant C M, Moore K H, *et al.* Calculating the direct costs of urinary incontinence: a new test instrument. *British Journal of Urology* 1999; **83**(6):596–606.

17 Kobelt G Economic considerations and outcome measurement in urge incontinence. *Urology* 1997; **50**(6A):100–7.

18 Wagner T H & Hu T-W Economic costs of urinary incontinence in 1995. *Urology* 1998; **51**(3):355–61.

19 Department of Health *Agenda for action on incontinence.*DOH, London 1991.

20 McGrother C, Resnick M, Yalla S V, *et al.* Epidemiology and etiology of urinary incontinence in the elderly. *World Journal of Urology*, 1991; **16**(1):S3–S9.

21 Ouslander J G & Briskewitz R Disorders of micturition in the ageing patient. *Advances in Internal Medicine*, 1989; **37**(2):197–8.

22 Button D, Roe B, Webb C, *et al.* Consensus guidelines – continence promotion and management by the primary health care team. Whurr Publishers Ltd, London 1998.

23 Royal College of Physicians *Incontinence – causes, management and provision of services*. RCP, London 1995.

24 Agency for Health Care Policy and Research, *Urinary incontinence in adults: acute and chronic management.* Clinical Practice Guideline, No. 2., 1996 update, AHCPR, US. Dept. of Health and Human Services.

25 Fantl J A, Wyman J F, McClish D K, *et al.*, Efficacy of bladder training in older women with urinary incontinence. *American Journal of Obstetrics & Gynaecology* 1991; **265**(5):609–13.

26 Malone-Lee J Recent developments in urinary incontinence in late life *Physiotherapy* 1994; **80**(3):133–4.

27 Cardozo L Urinary incontinence in women: do we have anything new to offer? *British Medical Journal* 1991; **303**(6815):1453–57.

28 Ouslander J G Causes, assessment, and treatment of incontinence in the elderly. *Urology*, 1990; **36**(4):25–35.

29 Brocklehurst J C Urinary incontinence in the community – analysis of a MORI poll. *British Medical Journal*, 1993; **306**(6881):832–4.

30 Cheater F, Lakhani M, & Cawood C *Audit protocol: assessment of patients with urinary incontinence.* CT14. Eli Lilly National Clinical Audit Centre, Leicester 1998.

31 Button D, *et al.* op. cit.

32 Fonda D, Benvenuti F, Castleden M, *et al.* Management of incontinence in older people. In Abrams P, Khoury S, & Wein A (Eds) *Incontinence* pp.731–3. 1st

International Consultation on Incontinence, World Health Organization and International Union Against Cancer 1999.

33 O'Brien J, Austin M, Seths P, *et al.* Urinary incontinence: prevalence, need for treatment, and effectiveness of intervention by nurse. *British Medical Journal.* 1991; **303**:1308–12.

34 The Multinational Tracking Survey *Overactive bladder problems – summary of key findings.* Sifo Research and Consulting AB, Pharmacia and Upjohn Ltd, Milton Keynes 1998.

35 Brocklehurst J C (1993), op. cit.

36 Button D, Roe B, Webb C, *et al. Consensus guidelines – continence promotion and management by the primary health care team.* Whurr Publishers Ltd, London 1998.

37 AHCPR (1996), op. cit.

38 Continence Foundation *A brief guide to urinary incontinence.* Continence Foundation, London 1998.

39 AHCPR (1996), op. cit.

40 Henderson J S & Taylor K H Age as a variable in an exercise program for the treatment of simple urinary stress incontinence. *J. Obstet. Gynecol Neonatal Nurs* 1987; **July/August**:266–72.

41 Burns P A, Pranikoff K, Nochajski T H, *et al.* A comparison of effectiveness of biofeedback and pelvic muscle exercise treatment of stress incontinence in older community-dwelling women. *Journal of Gerontology* 1993; **48**(4):M167–M174.

42 Wells T J, Brink C A, Diokno A C, *et al.* Pelvic muscle exercise for stress urinary incontinence in elderly women. *Journal of American Geriatricians Society* 1991; **39**(8): 785–91.

43 Bo K, Talseth T, & Holme I Single blind, randomised controlled trial of pelvic floor exercises, electrical stimulation, vaginal cones, and no treatment in management of genuine stress incontinence in women. *British Medical Journal,* 1999; **318**(7182): 487–94.

44 AHCPR (1996), op. cit.

45 Bo K, *et al* (1999), op. cit.

46 Burns, P A *et al.* (1993) op. cit.

47 Fonda D, *et al.* (1999), op. cit.

48 Winder A Intermittent self-catheterisation. In Roe BH (ed) *Clinical nursing practice. the promotion and management of continence* (1st ed.), pp 157–76. Prentice Hall, London 1992.

49 Oakeshott P & Hunt G M Intermittent self-catheterization for patients with urinary incontinence or difficulty emptying the bladder. *British Journal of General Practice.* 1992; **42**(359):253–5.

50 Wagg A & Malone-Lee J The management of urinary incontinence in the elderly. *British Journal of Urology* 1998; **82**(1):11–7.

51 Thuroff JW, et al. Medical treatment and medical side-effects in urinary incontinence in the elderly. *World Journal of Urology* 1998; **16**(1):S48–S61.

52 Pearson B D & Kelber S Urinary iIncontinence: treatments, interventions, and outcomes. *Clinical Nurse Specialist*, 1996; **10**(4):177–82.

53 James J, Sawczuk D, & Merrett S The effects of chronic caffeine consumption on urinary incontinence in psychogeriatric inpatients. *Psychology and Health*, 1989; **3**:297–305.

54 Gilbert R M Caffeine consumption. In Spiller G A (ed) *The methylxanthine beverages and foods: chemistry, consumption and health effects*, pp. 185–214. Alan R Liss, New York 1984.

55 McKinm E M & McKim W A Caffeine: how much is too much? *Canadian Nurse*, 1993; **89**(11):19–22.

56 Button D, et al., op. cit.

57 Pengelly A W & Booth A A prospective trial of bladder training as a treatment for detrusor instability. *British Journal of Urology*, 1980; **52**:463–6.

58 Burgio KL Behavioral training for stress and urge incontinence in the community. *Gerontology* 1990; **36**(**2**):27–34.

59 O Brien J (1991), op. cit.

60 Button D, et al. (1998), op. cit.

61 Robinson D, McClish D, Wyman J, Comparison between urinary diaries completed with and without intensive patient instructions. *Neurourological Urodynamics* 1996; **15**(2):143–8.

62 Wagg A & Malone-Lee J (1998), op. cit.

63 James M & Abrams P The drug treatment of urinary incontinence, *Prescriber* (1998); **9**(20):51–68.

64 Wagg A & Malone-Lee J (1998), op. cit.

65 James M & Abrams P (1998), op. cit.

66 James M & Abrams P (1998), op. cit.

67 Appell R A Clinical efficacy and safety of tolterodine in the treatment of overactive bladder: A pooled analysis. *Urology* 1997; **50**(6A):90–96.

68 James M & Abrams P (1998), op. cit.

69 Halaska M, Dorschner W, & Frank M Treatment of urgency and incontinence in elderly patients with propiverine hydrochloride. *Neurourological Urodynamics* 1994; **13**:428–38.

70 Chapple C R, Parkhouse H, Gardner G et al. Double-blind, placebo-controlled, cross-over study of flavoxate in the treatment of idiopathic detrusor instability. *British Journal of Urology* 1990; **66**(5):491–4.

71 Cardozo L Discussion: the effect of estrogens. *Urology* 1997; **50**(6A):85.

72 Stapleton A & Stamm W E Prevention of urinary tract infection. *Infectious Diseases Clinic of North America* 1997; **11**(3):719–33.

73 Cardozo L, Benness C, & Abbott D Low-dose oestrogen prophylaxis for recurrent urinary tract infections in elderly women. *British Journal of Obstetrics and Gynaecology,* 1998; **105**(4):403–7.

74 Continence Foundation, op. cit.

75 Lagro-Janssen R & Van Weel C Long-term effect of treatment of female incontinence in general practice. *British Journal of General Practice* 1998; **48**(436):1735–8.

76 Thomas G B Is there anyone else out there? *Nursing Times* 1987; **83**(21):32.

77 Ness W Silent problem. *Nursing Times.* 1994; **90**(36):67–70.

78 Kamm M A Obstetric damage and faecal incontinence. *Lancet.* 1994; **344**(8924):730–3.

79 Nelson R, Norton N, Cautley E, *et al.* Community-based prevalence of anal incontinence. Journal of the American Medical Association 1995; **274**(7):559–61.

80 Perry SI, Shaw C, Mensah C W, *et al.* and the MRC Incontinence Study Team *The prevalence of faecal incontinence in a community-based population.* Proceedings of the British Geriatrics Society Spring Meeting, Edinburgh 1998.

81 Petticrew M, Watt I, & Sheldon T *Systematic review of the effectiveness of laxatives in the elderly.* Executive Summary, Vol. 13. NHS Research and Development Health Technology Assessment Programme 1998.

82 Petticrew M, *et al.*, op. cit.

83 Wald A Constipation and faecal incontinence in the elderly. *Seminars in Gastrointestinal Disease,* 1994; **5**(4):179–88.

84 Whitehead W E, Drinkwater D, Chesking L J, *et al.* Constipation in the elderly living at home. Definition, prevalence, and relationship to lifestyle and health status. *Journal of the American Geriatricians Society* 1989; **37**(5):423–9.

85 Thompson W G, Creed F , Drossman D A , *et al.* Functional bowel disease and functional abdominal pain. *Gastroenterol Int.* 1992; **5**(2):75–91.

86 O'Keefe E A, Tally N J, Zinsmeister A J *et al.* Bowel disorders impair functional status and quality of life in the elderly: a population-based study. *J. Gerontol. A. Biol. Sci. Med. Sci.* 1995; **50**(4):184–9.

87 Wolfson C R, Barker J C, & Mitteness L S Constipation in the daily lives of frail elderly people. *Archives Family Medicine.* 1993; **2**:853–8.

88 Petticrew *et al.*, op. cit.

89 Goke M, Ewe K, Donner K *et al.* Influence of loperamide and loperamide oxide on the anal sphincter: a manometric study. *Diseases of the Colon & Rectum.* 1992; **35**(9):857–61.

90 Glickman S & Kamm M A Bowel dysfunction in spinal cord injury patients. *Lancet.* 1996; **347**(9016):1651–3.

91 Lorish T R , Sandin K J , Roth E J *et al.* Stroke rehabilitation 3. *Archives of Physical & Medical Rehabilitation* 1994; **75**(5):S47–51.

92 British National Formulary *Nurse Prescribers Formulary*. British Medical Association and Royal Pharmaceutical Society of Great Britain, London 1999.

93 Anthony B *The provision of continence supplies by NHS Trusts.* Unpublished report to Incontact, London 1998.

94 Cheater F., Lakhani M and Cawood C (1998), *Audit protocol: assessment of patients with urinary incontinence.* CT14 Eli Lilly National Clinical Audit Centre, Leicester.

95 Royal College of Physicians. *Promoting continence : clinical audit scheme for the management and promotion of urinary and faecal incontinence.* RCP London

96 Brocklehurst J (Chairman) (1999), *Health Outcome Indicators: Urinary Incontinence.* Report of a Working Group of the Department of Health, The National Centre for Health Outcomes Development, Oxford.

CHAPTER NINE

Depression, anxiety, and dementia

Old age brings plenty of problems. As we age we may face ill health, disability, dependency in ourselves or our spouse, problems with our housing, growing fear of our own vulnerability to crime, the desolation of social isolation and loneliness, and lower incomes. Our families give us other problems to worry about – separation, illness, failure, tragedy – and may not be willing or able to help us when we need them. Later life's a problem list, and then you die!

Looked at that way, depression and anxiety in old age become understandable, even 'normal' responses to declining faculties and dwindling resources. Dementia then becomes the cruellest way of outliving yourself, from which those of sound mind (even if not body) recoil in horror. Professionals and public alike can turn away from such problems, fatalistically attributing them to ageing because they believe that so little can be done.

Reality is very different from this grim scenario, although the perceptions of professionals working in primary care can be stubbornly but understandably stereotyping. We have concentrated experience of illness and disability, of the limited resources with which we can respond to growing demand, of our relative powerlessness to change the course of events, and of the sometimes wider gap between our understanding and practice, and existing scientific knowledge. The purpose of this chapter is to close that gap and reduce the sense of powerlessness experienced by primary care practitioners by describing the character and consequences of three common mental health problems of later life – depression, anxiety, and dementia – and the uncommon but serious issues of psychosis in old age.

Depression

Depression is the commonest psychiatric disorder in later life, with population studies showing that 10–15% of the population aged 65 or more suffer with significant depressive symptoms.[1] Only a small minority of depressed older individuals with significant symptoms receive treatment or referral, even though their general practitioners frequently recognize their depressed state.[2] Symptoms of depression in older people are associated with disability and with anxiety (see below), impeding easy recognition and complicating responses. The failure of primary care clinicians to act on a condition which they recognize, and the difficulties in conceptualizing the origins and course of late-life depression, are issues which have run through debates about ageing and mental health for the last 20 years, with few signs of resolution. Both GPs and hospital doctors have been criticized for their tendency to miss depression in their patients, but as we shall see the presentation and pattern of depression in older people in the community are so complex, and the uncertainties about the effectiveness of intervention so great that underdiagnosis is assured. Late-life depression is perhaps the best example of the limitations of the biomedical model of health and illness, and of the weakness of the idea of evidence-based practice, but it also reveals the scope for innovation in the community.

Conventional medical wisdom states that depression in later life is under-estimated, underdiagnosed, and undertreated. Its significance is under-estimated because:

- depressed people over the age of 65 are four times more likely to commit suicide than younger people (see below)
- depression in later life is associated with high use of both medical and social services
- depression particularly affects those older people caring for others.

It appears to be underdiagnosed because community studies show consistent underdocumenting of depression in medical records when compared with depression prevalence, and it is undertreated because:

- not all of those who have severe depression diagnosed are treated
- depressed older people are likely to be treated for anxiety (or physical symptoms like pain) rather than with antidepressants or psychological therapies – even though the commonest drugs used for suicide by self-poisoning amongst older people are painkillers and sleeping tablets or tranquillizers.

There appear to be persuasive clinical, social, and economic reasons for wanting to defeat depression, but how can primary care workers approach this when working with older people? Most older patients with depression consult their GP with a variety of physical and psychological symptoms. Continuity of care can provide a base from which to provide long-term care and commitment, and treatment can be given in a more familiar environment without stigmatizing the patient,[3] so recognition and management in primary care seems appropriate. However, recognition of depression in later life can be a problem in the community because the typical features of depressed mood or sadness may not be evident, or may be masked by anxiety, cognitive disturbance, or somatic complaints.[4] Sleep disturbance, failure to care for oneself, withdrawal from social life, unexplainable somatic symptoms, or hopelessness about a co-existing physical disorder may be the clues to depression, which might be best understood by both patient and practitioner as a physical disorder with emotional symptoms and an unclear biochemical basis.[5]

How can we sort out the complexity of late-life depression? One way to approach this is to consider the common diagnostic problems we encounter. Most older people with depression symptoms fall into the 'dysphoria' or 'demoralization syndrome' group where the appropriateness of the clinical label of depression may be contested by the patient and their family, often because the depression is associated with other problems, and where the effectiveness of treatments is unknown. Only a minority have severe depression which is clearly amenable to treatment. The specialist's perception of depression may not be helpful for those working with older people in the community because it explains neither the failure of conventional treatments to 'cure' depression, nor the paradoxical worldwide increase in suicide rates[6] alongside the apparent fall in depression prevalence,[7] when standard diagnostic criteria (like those of DSM1V or ICD10) are used.

'Minor depression'

The form of depression in later life that is characterized by variability of symptoms (and sometimes the dominance of anxiety), somatization, and an association with disability has acquired many names – 'demoralization syndrome', 'atypical depression', 'masked depression', 'subsyndromal depression', amongst others.[8] Because this form of depression falls outside the (specialist) criteria for major depression, it is also sometimes labelled 'minor depression', although this description is far from accurate and useful.

'Minor depression' in the community is:

- found amongst iller, older people
- associated with functional impairment, which may wax and wane in synchrony with depressive symptoms
- associated with cognitive impairment
- linked to later major depression
- associated with social and family impairment
- associated with higher death rates from all causes.

The adverse events associated with 'minor depression' occur as frequently as they do with 'major depression', making its identification seem necessary even if this is complicated by its overlap with other mental state disturbances (like dementia) and with organic mood syndromes (both endocrine and drug-induced). However, whilst screening for depression in older adults in British general practice, using a validated screening instrument, does yield more cases than clinical judgment reveals, once again identification does not seem to lead to treatment.[9] Feedback to primary care physicians about missed depression improved recognition, but did not alter management, in a similar American study.[10] The general practitioners in these studies may have been categorizing their patients by treatability, and not initiating any form of therapy or referral for those with 'minor depression' for whom they had no obvious treatment.

GPs faced with this complexity will tend to use pattern recognition and problem-solving logic pathways in an attempt to assist their patients. If the patterns learned by the GP, either formally through education or informally through experience, are less complex than the reality some other problem will be 'recognized' – anxiety, insomnia, or physical symptoms. Action will then be taken to solve these problems, even if the medication prescribed may not be appropriate for depression.

Anxiety and depression

How can primary care workers distinguish between depression overlaid by anxiety symptoms, and anxiety alone? Is there such a thing as uncomplicated anxiety in later life, or is all anxiety manifested by older people a sign of depression until proved otherwise? Does anxiety in old age develop into depression, over time, as some research suggests?[11] These are conceptual and diagnostic problems similar to those around subsyndromal depression, and equally in need of investigation. This need for knowledge is not academic because the presence or absence of anxiety symptoms in depression influences the outcome of symptoms, whilst phobic anxiety prompts well-intentioned but inappropriate home care for avoidant older people. Individuals with mixed anxiety and depression seem more likely to discontinue antidepressant medication, less likely to respond if they continue,[12] and likely to have shorter remissions even when treatment works[13] than depressed older patients without anxiety symptoms. Phobic anxiety in the absence of disabling physical problems may be the underlying cause of individuals becoming housebound in 20% of cases.[14]

Anxiety appears to be common in later life, with up to 10% of community-dwelling older adults meeting criteria for an anxiety disorder.[15] Anxiety symptoms are the commonest co-morbidity with depression,[16] and the majority of older people identified as having generalized anxiety disorder (GAD) also have depression symptoms.[17] Phobic anxiety, particularly amongst older women, is also common, affecting between 5% and 10% of the population aged 65 and over.[18] However, anxiety symptoms are also part of normal experience, and clinicians walk 'a fine line between pathologizing a healthy response and failing to recognize neurotic dysfunction'.[19] Symptoms and signs of anxiety may be somatic, cognitive or behavioural:

- **somatic** – palpitations, dry mouth, urinary frequency, dizziness, paraesthesia, difficulty breathing and hyperventilation, nausea, tremor, chest tightness, pallor, sweating, and cold skin
- **cognitive** – nervousness, feeling of dread, distractability, inability to relax, apprehension, panic, insomnia, and irritability
- **behavioural** hyperactivity, pressured speech, seeking reassurance, repetitive activity, phobias, and startle responses.

Individuals developing either depression or dementia may present with these anxiety symptoms, as can older people with thyroid disorders and subacute delirium secondary to infection, drug toxicity, electrolyte imbalance, and dehydration.

In situations where there is no underlying depression, dementia, or delirium, treatment options are bounded by the hazards of medication on one hand and the uncertain efficacy of psychological treatments on the other. Doctors prescribe, but medication for anxiety in later life is even more problematic than in younger people. Benzodiazepines are poorly metabolized, accumulation is associated with falls, confusion, and respiratory depression, and unsupported withdrawal may precipitate rebound anxiety or confusional states. Tricyclic antidepressants may induce urinary retention, oversedation and confusion, even at so-called subtherapeutic doses, whilst beta-blockers can precipitate cardiac failure, asthma, and depression, or interact with other medication, particularly calcium channel-blockers.[20]

Psychological approaches to treatment of anxiety symptoms may seem to offer more appropriate first-line therapy than current medication, but their effectiveness is unclear, and a widespread if inaccurate view that older people have little insight and are unable to deal with their problems in psychological terms may limit the options made available. We have tried to show that exactly the opposite is true in the discussion of health perceptions in Chapter 1 and of responses to disability in Chapter 5. The techniques that can be deployed include relaxation methods, cognitive behavioural approaches such as guided imagery, systematic desensitization and re-attribution, and family therapies.[20] Whilst the evidence base for these methods is slight, they may offer some scope for intervention with the phobic older person seeking (and getting) increased but inappropriate support at home from family, neighbours, and community services. Fear of street crime, for example, is common in the older generation, but there is no reason to believe that a chronic state of fear with disabling generalized avoidance behaviour that is dismissed euphemistically as 'nervousness' or 'loss of confidence' is a normal or inevitable consequence of growing old.[17]

Depression, illness, and disability

We first met Mrs D. in Chapter 1. Aged 91, she lives alone in a third-floor, one-bedroom flat in a small, relatively modern block of flats. Widowed for 20 years, she has a daughter (in her sixties) who lives 35 miles away, and one or two local friends whom she sees regularly each week. A neighbour helps her with shopping, and brings her to the practice from time to time. Travelling is a real struggle for her.

She is partially sighted (because of macular degeneration), and is just able to see the outlines of people and things, but no detail. She cannot watch television or read, but enjoys listening to the radio and talking books, even though she is moderately deaf. She had a myocardial infarction seven years ago, and has had cardiac failure since, causing progressively worsening exertional breathlessness and swelling of the ankles and calves. Her GP has recently asked her to take ACE inhibitor medication, but she declined on the grounds that she 'had enough medicines already'. She has had hypertension for at least 15 years and takes diuretics for this, and for her heart failure, frusemide (40mg, two each morning). Her BP control is reasonably good, with average pressures of 170/90. Her BMI is 31. When she complained about forgetfulness her doctor checked her cognitive function with the mini-Mental State examination, on which she scored 28 out of 30, failing only on the written responses.

Recently she was admitted by her GP to the local hospital with a painful, white left leg. The GP rightly thought she had an ischaemic leg, and this was confirmed on angiography, but the occlusion of arteries was too extensive and too distal to be corrected surgically, in the opinion of the vascular surgeons. To her GP's surprise, her limb pain has decreased despite the lack of treatment and she needs only regular co-proxamol (two, three times daily).

Bronchitis has been a regular problem over the years, occurring almost every autumn and winter. Last year she had episodes of wheezing in the summer, and was prescribed salbutamol by inhaler, together with a volumatic. Each autumn she attends for an influenza immunization. When she visits her GP she is jolly, describes herself as 'pretty good, all in all', and adds 'I mustn't grumble, there are many worse off than me'. Invariably she apologizes for wasting the doctor's time.

Everyone who has worked in primary care has met Mrs D., just as we have met depressed older people without major disabilities or illnesses. Why does she retain an optimistic and cheerful approach when others do not, and why are most older people with disabilities not depressed? The epidemiological answers about associations between disabilities, illness, and depression symptoms are only a slight help because an explanatory model of depression is needed to guide intervention. Here we run out of strong evidence, largely because of the paucity of longitudinal studies of depression in the community.[21] The association between poor health and depression appears to be greater for those aged 75 and over, and for men, than for younger old people as a whole, and for women. Subjective measures of ill health such as pain or self-rating of health are more strongly related to depression than are more objective measures of illness or disability such as the number of chronic diseases or the degree of functional limitation.[22] Nearly a third of older people with four or more medical problems are depressed, compared with one in 20 of those without a significant illness,[23] and the prevalence of depression amongst patients with poor physical health attending their GP is twice that of healthy attenders.[24] For those who work in the community such research findings intuitively make sense, but they are also hard to explain.

We can hypothesize about three explanations:[25]

(1) depressive disorder that is a clear reaction to illness or disability, or its treatment, and which fluctuates with the severity of the illness
(2) depression which preceeds the illness or disability, but which shares an origin with it (e.g. a life event such as bereavement)
(3) depressive disorder which precedes the onset of the physical problems and which may be responsible for them (a somatization disorder).

Clinically it is not easy to distinguish depression symptoms from symptoms of illness or disability – for example, tiredness, loss of appetite, and weight loss can be features of many illnesses as much as they can be components of depression. Nevertheless, making the distinction may matter because depression in later life is associated with higher than expected morbidity, disability, and mortality from a wide range of natural causes.[26] One large-scale community study has shown that the relative risks of both all-cause mortality and cardiovascular mortality are highest in depressed individuals with established heart disease, but are also elevated in those with no evidence of cardiovascular pathology at entry to the study.[27] Depression is one of the main risk factors for sudden death up to one year after myocardial infarction, after adjustment for other risk factors,[28] and also predicts a poorer outcome after life-threatening illness such as subarachnoid haemorrhage, pulmonary embolism, or bleeding peptic ulcer, even allowing for illness severity.[29]

A model of late-life depression

How can primary care doctors and nurses working in conditions of high demand, short contacts with patients, and complex presentations of problems deal with all the uncertainties surrounding depression in later life? Without a workable conceptual framework for late-life depression, its symptoms are easy to dismiss as normal for the patient's age, or understandable in the context of illness or disability. Fortunately psychology and sociology come to our aid with a hypothetical model of late-life depression[30] that fits the available epidemiological and observational evidence, and offers a range of domains in which interventions can be made systemically. Figure 9.1 shows how depression may emerge in later life, and what its effects may be.

A systemic approach to late-life depression allows multiple responses to a problem with many dimensions, with therapeutic interventions tailored to individuals. The following case is an example.

Mr A. (whom we also first met in Chapter 1) had a stroke affecting the left side of his body not long after his 74th birthday, and within a few weeks of moving to a new flat in a new town. The woman with whom he had lived for 10 years left him the next day, saying that she could not care for him. After a brief hospital admission where rehabilitation was started he made a good functional recovery, aided by visits from the community physiotherapist, modification to his (ground-floor) flat by the OT from social services, and home help support from social services.

He remained distraught at the loss of the woman he still loved, and frustrated by his inability to do all the things he needed and wanted to do around the flat, and in his tiny garden. During visits to his GP he would sometimes weep copiously, but he always refused any medication for his depressed mood, sleeplessness, and lack of energy. Although he often said that he saw no point in going on, he slowly became more socially active, finally joining an exercise class at the local gym and a luncheon club where he got 'good food and some company'.

He began to complain about increasingly troublesome prostate symptoms, and was found to have prostatic cancer. His urologist carried out a transurethral prostatectomy and proposed a long course of anti-androgen treatment, which Mr A. accepted. His mood worsened with recurrence of crying bouts, he left the exercise class because, he said, he was 'embarrassed at being with so many old women', and he became increasingly hopeless and neglectful of his home and himself. Although his prostatic symptoms improved significantly, all investigations

Figure 9.1 *Antecendents and consequences of depression in later life.*

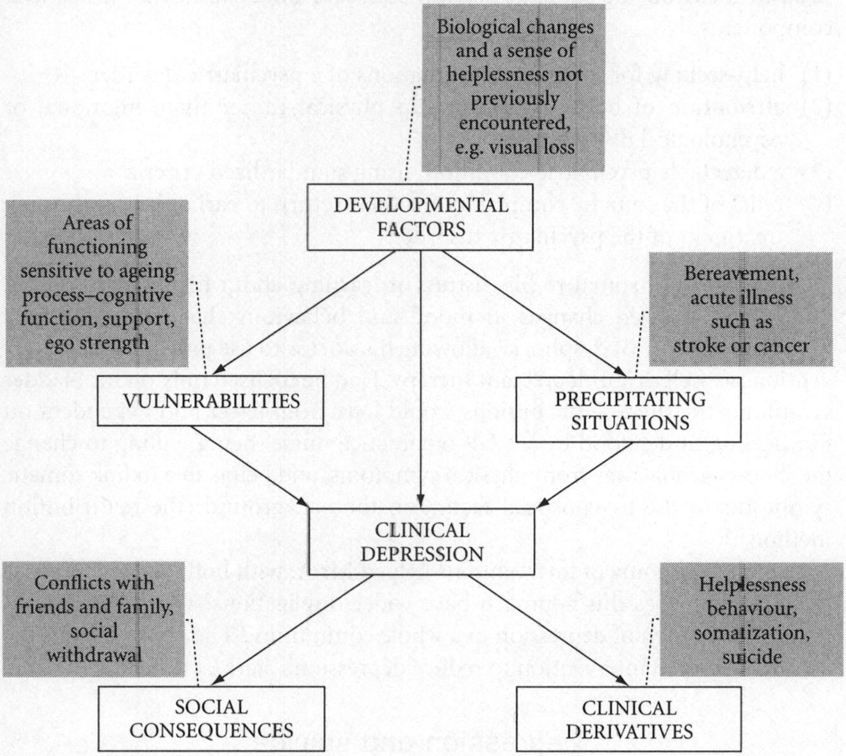

failed to show metastatic spread of the tumour, and his prostate-specific antigen (PSA) remained within the normal range, he was always worried that he was not being told the whole truth and that the cancer was spreading. He also became involved in the problems of an equally old neighbour, whose brother had died tragically and unexpectedly, causing immense distress to his surviving family. The depressed and the bereaved bickered and argued constantly, each telling the other to 'get over it' and 'pull yourself together'.

Although he was reluctant to consider antidepressant medication Mr A. did agree that his depression needed attention and consulted an old-age psychiatrist, on whose recommendation he commenced fluoxetine. His GP was able to obtain intensive bereavement counselling for the neighbour (who was also a patient of the practice), and also copied all Mr A.'s medical records so that he could see the correspondence about his prostate tumour and all the results of tests. The concerns about cancer faded away, Mr A. resumed his exercise class after a three-month break, but the two neighbours continued to quarrel, each accusing the other of not looking after himself properly.

Somatization

Making sense of physical symptoms and teasing out physical illness from depression is not necessarily easy. When are patients ill, and when do they exhibit depressive somatization or a somatization disorder? To answer this we need to focus on the somatisation process, and understand that it has four components:[31]

(1) help-seeking for somatic manifestations of a psychiatric disorder
(2) attribution of bodily symptoms to physical rather than emotional or psychological disturbance
(3) a detectable psychiatric condition, using standardized criteria
(4) relief of the somatic complaints (or their return to earlier levels) through treatment of the psychiatric disorder.

Mr A. did not somatize his distress at learning about his prostate cancer, but instead showed changes in mood and behaviour that amounted to a 'psychologization' of dysphoria, allowing his doctor to use psychological interventions as well as antidepressant therapy. Had he focused only on his bladder symptoms the therapeutic options would have been fewer and dependent on him feeling understood by his GP or practice nurse, being willing to change the illness agenda away from physical symptoms, and being able to link somatic symptoms to the psychosocial factors in the background (the reattribution method).[32]

A mixed economy of interventions helped Mr A. with both of his depressive episodes, but does this approach have wider implications? Can it be used to reduce the burden of depression in a whole community? The greatest test is the ability of tailored intervention to reduce depression's starkest outcome, suicide.

Depression and suicide

Depression is clearly the psychiatric condition most often linked to suicide among older adults.[33] High and rising rates of suicide among older adults – particularly men – are a worldwide phenomenon,[34,35] and the increasing incidence of depression in recent cohorts portends ominously for future generations of older adults. Those particularly at risk are older white men, living alone, with depression associated with multiple physical symptoms and sleep disturbance, who also have other significant physical illness, who have been bereaved recently, and who have made previous suicide attempts.[21] Identification of those at greatest risk and the pursuit of a systemic approach to their medical and social care appears to be effective. In an important Scandinavian study, Rutz and colleagues evaluated a community-wide approach to prevention of suicide through an intervention directed at general practitioners.[36] The investigators attempted to educate all GPs on an island in Sweden regarding suicide and depression in late life, and found a significant decline in suicide rates on the island when compared to trends in the rest of Sweden. The rates for the island and for the rest of Sweden were comparable for 17 years, but declined on the island following the intervention. While there are difficulties in interpreting the study with regard to cause and effect, the findings suggest that a sustained effort centred in general practice can lead to prevention of depression and suicide among older adults.

How can we put all of this into practice? We suggest three headings for consideration – organization, education, and intervention. Firstly, we should capitalize on the existing patterns of services used by the depressed elderly through which to improve the capacity of the primary health care network to recognize and respond to these patients. This is an argument against dedicated programmes and special teams designed to bypass the problems of under-detection and under-response to late-life depression, and in favour of improving the performance of what we already possess – the existing, elaborate networks of general practice, community health services, and social care.

Enhancing pattern recognition for late-life depression amongst primary care workers with a more complex understanding of depression in later life and the promotion of a systemic approach to intervention appears to be appropriate and may justify the 'defeat depression' campaigning approach to professional education and practice. This is where the specialist outreach team has a dual role, by using its responses to the complexities of diagnosing and managing depression in *some* older patients to educate generalists who work with *all* older people. We will discuss the operational implications of skill transfer in such a potentially synergistic relationship in Chapter on teamwork.

Depression has social and historic origins in older people, just as it does in younger adults, and social responses – through richer social networks, through opportunities for social activity, through work, through regular physical exercise – as well as psychological approaches may offer just the 'treatments' that GPs lack. There is a strong sense of the importance of non-medical treatment options in general practice, as the growth of counselling, rehabilitation, and alternative medicine in practice settings shows. The key to improving the quality of care for depressed older people in the community lies with the idea of 'networking', a notion that has entered the vocabulary of general practice in the last five years. Networking – as opposed to its medical rival, 'referral' – is a social term implying dialogue and contact, and so takes us back to the discussion of communications between GPs and social workers in Chapters 2 and 3, and forward to the description of community-oriented primary care in Chapter 11.

Dementia

Dementia is not rare, but for the average GP it is an uncommon problem. About 8% of the population over 75 years of age will have some degree of dementia, so that a typical GP with 2000 patients, of whom about 130 are over 75, will know perhaps 10 or 11 affected individuals – although s/he may not know they have dementia. Given that the life expectancy of people with dementia is 5–10 years from diagnosis, a new diagnosis may be made only every year or so, against a background of between 6000 and 8000 consultations. Alzheimer's disease is the commonest form of dementia, accounting for two-thirds of cases overall, and its prevalence increases with advancing age. About 5% of people aged 65 and over have some form of dementia, with the prevalence rising to about 20% by 80 years and nearer one in three by 90. Alzheimer's disease costs the UK economy an estimated £1.5 billion per year.[37]

The dementias are therefore a growing challenge for primary care providers. With the increasing prevalence of the dementias in an ageing population[38] and the shift away from long-term institutional care, primary care workers find themselves dealing with increasing numbers of patients with dementia, and with their families and neighbours.[39] General practitioners and their teams are uniquely situated in the British system of health care to achieve early diagnosis and optimal management in the community of dementia, yet there is evidence of underdiagnosis, under-response to established dementia, and inadequate management[40,41] in Britain as there is in other countries.[42,43] The majority of respondents to a national survey of British GPs felt inadequately trained in the diagnosis and management of dementia,[44] but there is little evidence of its provision despite the perceived need to reconfigure interprofessional education towards future tasks.[45]

This gap in knowledge and skills appears to be an international phenomenon, there being wide variations in knowledge about dementia amongst GPs,[46] with memory impairment being the most commonly recognized symptom[47] in an otherwise limited conception of the disease. GPs often believe that they have little to offer dementia patients,[48] experience explaining the diagnosis of dementia as being particularly difficult,[49] and sometimes consider that giving a diagnosis does more harm than good[4] because relatives do not want to be confronted with this reality.[50] Studies of relatives of dementing patients report that physicians are reluctant to make a diagnosis[51,52] and tend to minimize problems,[6] whilst focusing on the hopeless nature of dementia.[53] To remedy this situation an educational agenda has been proposed on the basis of a review of existing studies,[3] and suggests that attention should be paid to: (i) diagnosis; (ii) screening instruments; (iii) referral criteria; (iv) carers' problems; and (v) information about support services.

Dementia does not have a typical 'textbook' character until it is advanced, and both the affected individual and near relatives and friends may disguise changes in memory, personality, and behaviour, consciously or unconsciously, so that the problem is not easily identified. Alzheimer's disease is much misunderstood, and its diagnosis and management are a challenge. In its early stages it is characterized by memory deficits and other changes in cognition, including some features of depression. Functional losses then appear, and in the later stages higher mental functions are lost so that the affected individuals suffer disorientation and loss of comprehension, the ability to calculate, learning capacity, language, and judgement. The personality begins to change, with emotional lability, disinhibition, and sometimes verbal or even physical aggression emerging as consistent features. At the end stage the individual with dementia loses almost all functional capacity, often becomes incontinent of urine and faeces, and may be unable to communicate with others in any way.

Alzheimer's disease:

- is a neurodegenerative disorder
- which produces cerebral atrophy, amyloid plaques, and neurofibrillary tangles in the brain
- with an asssociated acetylcholine deficiency
- and a gradual, progressive course, different from the step-wise course of vascular (multi-infarct) dementia
- which is chronic, unlike the sudden onset of confusional states due to infection or drug effects.

Differential diagnosis

As the dementing process proceeds, awareness of memory or other problems with cognition decreases so the patient becomes a less reliable witness. Carers' complaints about the memory of a family member are suggestive of dementia, whereas complaints of memory loss made by the patient suggest depression rather than dementia.[54] However, there is no classic presentation since one in three patients with dementia will also have features of either a depressive disorder or symptoms attributable to bereavement, or generalized anxiety, or an alcohol problem. Patients with Alzheimer's disease tend not to complain about physical symptoms, even when they have morbidity that should produce them, and somatic complaints can be a sign of depression. However, depression and dementia can co-exist in up to 40% of individuals with cognitive impairment, occurring mostly in the early stages of the dementing process and having an increased mortality. Treatment of the depression seems to be effective in terms of restoring some function and reducing psychological distress in up to 85% of those with both disorders.

Lewy body dementia is uncommon but presents with a different pattern of symptoms (Box 9.1). Patients with Lewy body dementia should not be treated with neuroleptic drugs because of a high risk of consequent acute illness and death.

Box 9.1 *Clinical pattern in Lewy body dementia (symptoms in order of frequency)*

- clouding of consciousness
- paranoid delusions
- complex visual hallucinations
- falls and 'collapses'
- depression symptoms
- auditory hallucinations

Delayed diagnosis

This complexity means that the changes of dementia may be attributed to other causes, especially early in the illness. Delay in the presentation and recognition of the dementia process can be due to:

- poor awareness of dementia characteristics amongst family members
- denial of the implications of changes in thinking and behaviour by family members, and by professionals
- high levels of respect for elderly relatives
- the attribution of both memory and functional loss to normal ageing
- and sometimes the negligible impact of early dementia on family life and family economics.

The triggers that start the process of recognition of dementia are commonly:

- important functional changes, such as not taking prescribed medication regularly
- behavioural disturbances, such as wandering or acting in a disinhibited way
- major loss of memory, such as losing the way home from the shops
- other cognitive and mood changes, such as the expression of paranoid ideas
- or crises – the revelatory moments when the spouse who has compensated so long for the failing memory or ability of their dementing partner has a stroke, or fractures their femur, and is admitted to hospital.

Both family members and professionals who have known the affected individual for some time may respond to the recognition of dementia with disbelief that such a process is underway, denial that the problem is dementia, sometimes with a search for another, more tolerable explanation, apprehension at the level of support that will be required for the individual and those around him or her, or fear of the illness.

Early detection

Early identification may be important for forward planning of care, for education of patients, families, and professional teams, and for mobilization of resources. Deterioration in four domains of daily activity is associated with cognitive impairment:

(1) managing medication
(2) using the telephone
(3) managing a budget
(4) using transport.

Cognitive function tests are useful adjuncts to clinical judgement and informant histories. The two most widely used are the Abbreviated Mental Test Score (AMTS) and the mini-Mental State Examination (MMSE). Both have advantages and disadvantages, and neither are diagnostic, they are simply suggestive of cognitive impairment. There is much to be gained by using whichever one is in current use by the geriatricians or old-age psychiatrists in your area.

Investigation

In a small proportion of patients with dementia there is an underlying pathology that, when treated, may result in some improvement in cognitive function – but not necessarily reversal of the dementing process. Co-morbidities to exclude when investigating possible dementia are:

- hypothyroidism (and, rarely, so-called 'apathetic hyperthyroidism')
- B_{12} deficiency
- hyperglycaemia
- hypocalcaemia (from hyperparathyroidism, sarcoidosis and myeloma)
- hypercalcaemia (from metastatic cancer)
- renal failure.

Brain tumours are rare causes of dementia-like syndromes, as is normal-pressure hydrocephalus (in which ataxia, urinary incontinence, and dementia are the classic triad), but families and dementia support groups may want these unlikely probabilities explored.

The minimum investigation list for an individual with suspected dementia should be:

- a full blood count
- renal function
- thyroid-stimulating hormone (TSH)
- calcium levels
- blood glucose.

Disclosing the diagnosis

This is the task that everyone finds most difficult, but it seems essential to carers that their anxieties about dementia are dealt with directly – one of the commonest complaints heard in voluntary organizations working with dementia sufferers and their families is 'nobody told us what was happening'. In general practice we have to balance our uncertainty about the diagnosis with the need to include it as a possibility that needs investigation. Discussion of the nature of the disease process, its course, and the palliative responses that can be made to it needs to happen earlier rather than later. False hopes about cures or even short-term improvements are as unhelpful as saying 'there is nothing that can be done'.

Management planning

Care of an individual with dementia requires different disciplines to work together. A management plan is important, shared across a multidisciplinary network that includes the main carers and local voluntary organizations. This plan should include:

- a needs assessment that includes co-morbidities, mental state, difficulties with activities of daily living, and behavioural problems, organized as a minimum data set that can be exchanged between disciplines
- support for carers, including information about legal rights and responsibilities (Box 9.2), financial help (Box 9.3), and driving (Box 9.4)
- a tailored follow-up programme, identifying a key worker and the responsibilities of other practice members
- referral criteria to different agencies, agreed locally
- specialist input on medication use, particularly with the new anti-dementia drugs that are emerging at the rate of two a year.

Box 9.2 *Legal issues in Alzheimer's disease*

Seek advice and background information on:

- enduring power of attorney
- Court of Protection and Public Office Trust
- guardianship.

Box 9.3 *Financial support*

The minimum benefit entitlement should be:

- disability living allowance care component (under 65)
- attendance allowance (65 and over)
- invalid care allowance for carers
- reduction in, or exemption from, council tax.

Box 9.4 *Driving*

The patient has a legal duty to inform the DVLA if diagnosed as having dementia. They may be given a Group 1 licence if there is no significant deterioration in time and space, and retention of insight and judgement, but an annual medical review is needed for renewal. The GP should inform the DVLA if the patient cannot understand this advice.

The key worker should be the first point of contact for the patient and carer, chosen with the patient and carer if possible, named and recorded in the medical and social care records, able to contact other relevant professionals, and able to nominate a deputy.

Behaviour disturbances

Behaviour disturbances in dementia can be a major source of stress for both family and professional carers, and need to be investigated carefully to tailor responses and avoid iatrogenesis. Wandering is associated with repeated falls and nocturnal wandering is predictive of institutionalization. Aggressive behaviour is associated with other underlying medical disorders, delusions or misidentifications, and the care setting and the attitudes of carers.

A malignant social psychology can undermine individuals with dementia, just when they are most vulnerable and in need of support, by objectifying, infantilizing, invalidating, overwhelming, or ignoring them (amongst other techniques).[55] Communication with the patient with dementia may be the key to both understanding and resolving behaviour disturbances, but it should hinge on four qualities:[56]

(1) self-esteem – is enhanced when the patient is recognized as a person
(2) agency – is confirmed when a gesture is converted into action
(3) social confidence – increases when the patient is welcomed
(4) hope – sustained when the stability of the social environment meets the confusion of dementia itself.

Wherever possible, underlying causes for behaviour disturbance should be managed before prescribing medication. Tranquillizer use to control behaviour disturbance should not be prescribed routinely, although short-term use of neuroleptic agents may be appropriate in crisis situations (unless Lewy body dementia is suspected). The expertise of community psychiatric nurses and old-age psychiatrists is invaluable in assessing and dealing with behaviour disorders.

Prescribing

Medication use in dementia is controversial because:

*   neuroleptics given for behaviour disturbance can precipitate falls and confusion without necessarily having a beneficial effect on behaviour
*   antidepressants in therapeutic dosages may have a significant effect on depression symptoms in early dementia, but need to be evaluated against explicit criteria such as activities of daily living, level of functioning, behaviour disturbance, and biological features of recent onset
*   donepezil may make a difference to cognitive function scores in mild to moderate Alzheimer's disease, but its impact on day-to-day functioning, quality of life, or overall clinical rating of dementia is not always significant. Its use in primary care cannot be supported on the current evidence of its efficacy. The basic cost to the NHS of a 12-week course of donepezil, at a starting dose of 5 mg was about £205 in 1999.

Carers

Family carers of patients with dementia experience prolonged strain, which may result in precipitate admission of the patient to hospital or other institution as well as contributing to physical and mental ill health in the carer. Primary care workers need to know that:

- support groups for dementia are valued by carers but may not reduce strain
- respite care provides carers with satisfaction but does not appear to alter their overall well-being
- depression is common in carers and is associated with behavioural problems and higher dependence in the patient and low income in the household, but not with the severity of the cognitive impairment itself
- acknowledging distress in carers and providing more information about dementia increases their satisfaction with services
- men carers complain less about the burden of caring, but experience it as much as women
- the stress of caring is not necessarily reduced by the institutionalization of the dementia sufferer.

Day care and packages of home care delay institutionalization, which is often prompted by a combination of carer stress, irritability or aggression, physical dependence, nocturnal wandering, and incontinence.

Support and information

The Alzheimers's Society provides information about all major causes of dementia and support for families with an individual with dementia through its 300 branches in England, Wales, and Northern Ireland. Alzheimer's Scotland provides a similar service.

Alzheimer's Society
Gordon House
10 Greencoat Place
London SW1P 1PH

Tel. 0207 306 0606

Alzheimer's Scotland
22 Drumheugh Gardens
Edinburgh EH3 7RN

Tel. 0131 243 1453

In summary, there are a number of features of dementia that make its identification and management difficult, especially in general practice. They are:

- the small number of individuals who develop dementia in any practice over a period of time
- the different ways in which dementia affects individuals and their families, sometimes making identification difficult
- the lack of an immediate, technical response to dementia
- the historic cultural difference between general practice and social services
- the emotional significance of dementia, especially in long-standing relationships between doctors and their patients.

Early detection and optimal management require the same teamworking/

networking approaches as outlined for depression. Primary care team members need to consider the following:

(1) Diagnosing and managing dementia is a complex task that needs a systematic approach.

(2) Brief screening instruments for cognitive loss can be useful aids to diagnosis, and informant accounts are essential.

(3) The task for primary care teams is a palliative one, involving appropriate investigation and treatments, collaborative and flexible working, and an active management style.

(4) Investigations for potentially remediable pathology contributing to the dementia should be carried out in general practice.

(5) Specialist help should be sought when there are uncertainties about the diagnosis – acute confusion is usually easy to distinguish from dementia but depression and dementia may co-exist, and Lewy Body disease, although rare, needs identification.

(6) Regular and detailed communication with the patient, the family, and other professionals is crucial to effective care.

(7) Local voluntary organizations like Alzheimer's Society branches can provide information and support for patients, their families, and their professional carers.

(8) Identifying a key worker, and establishing a mechanism for regular reviews of the management plan, are important aspects of good practice in dementia care.

(9) There is little evidence to support the use of donepezil in general practice, and specialist advice should be sought about prescribing both this drug and neuroleptics.

(10) Training of primary care teams in dementia management is useful because of the low incidence of the disease, the complexities of the disease processes, the distress they induce, and the range of different agencies that may be involved.

PCGs have a ready-made set of criteria for measuring the quality of care in dementia, and access to training materials. Dementia is a topic which tests the ability of different disciplines to collaborate and to work across the generalist/ specialist divide.

There are two useful training sources, suitable for practice-based learning or group work in vocational training and other continuing medical education:

• *Dementia in the Community: management strategies for general practice.* Alzheimer's Society (1995). Designed as a workbook and particularly useful for registrar training.

• *Action in Alzheimer's: practise-based learning pack.* Excerpta Medica UK, Reed Healthcare Communications, The Boulevard, Langford Lane, Kidlington, Oxford OX5 1GB. Designed around problem-solving approaches tested in multidisciplinary workshops across the UK in 1997.

Mr K., who is now 85, cared for his wife Margaret for seven years whilst her Alzheimer's disease progressed. He noticed at first that she was becoming forgetful, but neither he nor his daughters (who lived some distance away) thought much of this until she became unable to go shopping and began to have difficulties with her usual household chores. As the months passed Margaret did less and less, although she enjoyed visiting her family and especially liked to go to the local church club, which met most weekdays. A fellow church member escorted her there and back each day, whilst Mr K. got on with housework and went shopping. Her dementia became an issue for her GP when Mr K. developed acute bronchitis and took to his bed for a week, leaving a helpless, forgetful wife in charge of the home. The family intervened to manage the situation, but the diagnostic process began. A domiciliary visit by an old-age psychiatrist confirmed the GP's diagnosis of probable Alzheimer's disease. No abnormalities were found on blood tests, and Margaret K. remained cheerful but inactive. Mr K. refused any help from social services, saying that he would 'carry on as long as he could'. His daughters disagreed with his attitude to support but were unable to change his mind. The GP kept in touch with the family regularly by phone, and visited Mr and Mrs K. often, more to open a dialogue with Mr K.

When Margaret K began to wake her husband frequently at night to ask him the same questions repeatedly, and in an increasingly belligerent way, Mr K began to reconsider the situation. Her deterioration was rapid, and events overtook his plans to accept help at home. She was admitted to a nursing home after a brief inpatient stay on a geriatric ward, precipitated by a fall at home.

Margaret K died within two weeks of admission to institutional care, leaving her husband feeling guilty that he had allowed this relocation to occur. His family began to arrange for him to move into sheltered accommodation near them, but he continues to resist this idea, having been in favour of it before his wife's death. His GP continues to visit regularly, and keep in touch with the daughters by telephone. Mr K scored 27 out of 30 on the mini Mental State examination at a recent visit, but remains worried about his deteriorating memory.

We can sum up the diagnostic and management pathway for dementia in primary care in Figure 9.2.

Psychoses in later life – the scale of the problem

Psychotic disorders in old age are overshadowed by dementia and depression, both of which occur more commonly, but they are no less problematic for the primary care doctor or nurse to diagnose or manage. The research literature about late-onset psychoses that could guide practitioners is sparse compared with that for the commoner psychiatric disorders, and very small when compared with that for mental illness in younger people.[57] Yet everyone who has worked in general practice or community nursing will have encountered patients whose symptoms suggest a psychotic disorder, and who pose a difficult management problem. As the population ages, more older individuals will present with delusions, hallucinations, or marked hypochondriasis amongst a wide range of other symptoms. Psychosis in old age often needs specialist attention, both for diagnosis and for treatment, but its nature may

Figure 9.2 Pathway for diagnosis and management of dementia.

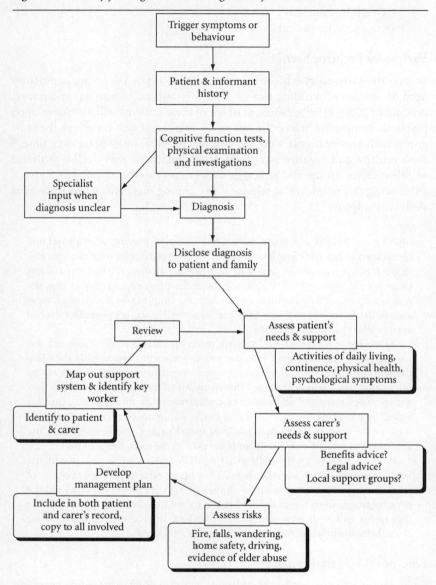

prevent or delay specialist referral, especially when paranoid features are present in the illness. The general practitioner confronted with it needs to understand the essentials of late-life psychoses in order to inform and advise families, brief other agencies working with the patient, and seek appropriate specialist support.

There are five major psychoses that affect older people:

(1) early-onset schizophrenia in its late stages
(2) late-onset schizophrenia

(3) delusional or paranoid disorders
(4) psychosis in dementia
(5) psychosis in depression.

Early-onset schizophrenia

In later life early-onset schizophrenia may affect up to 1% of the population aged 65 and over,[58] yielding two or three affected individuals in an 'average' practice of 2000 patients. Nine out of ten of these patients will have developed psychotic symptoms before the age of 45 years, and will represent the sub-group with schizophrenia whose symptoms remit or ameliorate over time.[59] Both positive and negative symptoms of schizophrenia may decline with age in this survivor group, and although social networks shrink (as with most of us as we age), the quality of relationships, coping mechanisms and practical skills may improve.[60]

> Miss L. had trained as a nurse, but stopped hospital nursing after a psychotic breakdown in her late twenties. However, with regular medication she was able to work as a private nurse, providing night-sitting services for frail but affluent older people. Although often deluded about the cause of everyday events, she was usually cheerful and worked energetically on simple tasks. She lived alone in a small flat but coped well with bills and household work, supported by a social worker who visited her regularly.
>
> At the age of 58 she retired from her work, saying that it was 'too much' for her, and it became apparent that she was experiencing increasingly disabling thought disorder. A new symptom appeared – repetitive stamping whilst sitting in her armchair – which distressed the occupants of the flat below, but after psychiatric assessment and adjustment of medication made no difference, this was solved by providing a thick cushion for her to stamp on. She remained cheerful most of the time, although now prone to mood swings, and developed a close and supportive relationship with an older man in the same block of flats.
>
> Increasing contact with both social services and a community psychiatric nurse was needed to maintain her in her home. Her high consumption of cigarettes led to the development of chronic obstructive airways disease, and she became progressively less mobile in her late sixties. She died at the age of 72 after setting fire to her duvet whilst smoking in bed, the recently installed smoke alarm being insufficient to prevent fatal smoke inhalation.

Late-onset schizophrenia

Only 3% of patients with schizophrenia develop their psychotic symptoms after the age of 60,[61] making late-onset schizophrenia an uncommon problem for primary care workers. The distinction may be academic, however, for the clinical features of early-and late-onset schizophrenia are similar, the only significant difference being fewer negative symptoms amongst older patients. Pre-morbid personality may influence the onset of schizophrenia in later life, with the following descriptions given by family members:[62]

- humourless
- solitary

- reserved
- hostile
- unsympathetic
- suspicious
- eccentric
- quarrelsome
- cold
- having odd religious views.

Mr L. arrived in Britain in the late 1950s from Jamaica at the age of 33, married soon after arrival, and had three children in rapid succession. His wife left him when the children were in their teens, saying he was impossible to live with, and the children also moved out of the family home as soon as they could, although they stayed in the neighbourhood and kept in contact with their father.

Always a critical man with few friends, he became increasingly reclusive after retirement, and spent his time writing immensely complicated, illustrated treatises on God and the Devil which filled sheets of paper or cardboard from margin to margin. His sleeping pattern became erratic, and his flat disorganized. He would watch the street from his window, talk to his children about people and vehicles spying on him, and from time to time abuse passers-by from a first-floor window.

The local mental health team were asked to see him at home, with his family, where he was suspicious and evasive, refusing all help and support. He was not considered a danger to himself or others, and his family were left to contain his psychopathology, with arms-length support from his GP and the team's community psychiatric nurse.

Delusional and paranoid disorders

Paranoia as a symptom is more common than late-onset schizophrenia, affecting 4% of the population over 65, but may be associated with it, or with dementia. It affects older women more than men. Paranoid symptoms are associated with previous personality disorder, hearing loss, immigrant status, and low socio-economic status.[63] There are also possible associations with physical or sexual abuse in early life, and not having had children.[64]

Mrs C. had not been seen by her GP for four years when the local social services department asked him to visit her. She was 78, lived alone, and had been annoying her neighbours by banging on the walls of her terraced house during the night and shouting accusations at them in the street by day.

When her GP visited he found the letterbox blocked with cloth, and at first was unable to get any response to the doorbell. A neighbour came to the rescue by standing on the back garden wall and tapping on Mrs C.'s window with a cane – she was very deaf, and had not heard her doorbell at all. She agreed to let the GP in, but first had to dismantle a barricade of poles and planks that she had constructed inside her front door.

The house was dilapidated, and there was little evidence of food or food preparation in the kitchen, although tomatoes were ripening on every window-sill in the house. Mrs C. explained that her neighbours were breaking in and stealing her clothes, and also using her bath to wash, although a thick layer of grime suggested that noone had used the bath for a long time. She described them in graphically abusive terms, and when pressed with questions about herself stopped speaking English, reverting instead to her first language, Hungarian.

A domiciliary visit by an old-age psychiatrist was requested, and to her GP's surprise she accepted admission to hospital – but only as a respite from her neighbours.

Psychosis in dementia

About one-third of patients with Alzheimer-type dementia develop psychotic symptoms, particularly persecutory delusions and visual rather than auditory hallucinations.[65] Visual or hearing impairment appears to increase the risk of developing psychotic symptoms in dementia, and those with a previous history of a psychiatric disorder are also at higher risk.[66] The greater the cognitive impairment in dementia, the more likely it is that psychotic symptoms will emerge.[67]

Miss N. had been 'in service' all her working life and described herself as 'a bit of a loner'. In her early eighties she became too frail to stay in the bedsitter that she had occupied for 20 years, and with social services help moved to warden-controlled accommodation nearby.

It became obvious after a short time that she was developing a dementing illness, and the level of support services available for her was increased to maintain her autonomy in her new home. The home helps and care assistants began to complain that she was becoming verbally abusive, and was accusing them of stealing her money and her few precious possessions. She began describing visits by non-existent people, and then struck a care assistant who was helping her to put her shoes on. The warden and community staff asked for her to be moved out of her accommodation to a nursing home.

Psychosis in depression

Persecutory and hypochondriacal delusions within a depressive disorder occur in only 1% of those over 65, whilst 20% of this age group have some depression symptoms, but delusions are associated with greater severity of depression and higher likelihood of referral to psychiatrists and admission to hospital.[68] Surprisingly, delusions associated with depression are not associated with a worse outcome, but do tend to persist through successive episodes of depression.[69] Depression in later life differs greatly in its presentation from depression in younger adults, with depressed mood being conspicuous by its absence whilst somatic complaints are prominent. The boundary between multiple physical complaints in an individual who does have arthritis, chronic lung disease, and depression and the overwhelming preoccupation with bodily symptoms which fit no pattern in the hypochondriacally deluded patient may be difficult to discern, explaining why referral and admission are more common for this group.

Mrs O. had had several episodes of depression treated in general practice during her life, had embarked on psychotherapy in her fifties, and had needed an admission to hospital with depression. In her late sixties her husband died from Parkinson's disease, and not long afterwards she developed low back pain associated with inexplicable tingling feelings all over, strange headaches, marked fluctuations in energy, and strange rashes that no one else could see. She fiercely denied that she was depressed, and offered an alternative explanation of her symptoms – she had contracted syphilis from a casual sexual encounter early in her marriage, had transmitted it to her husband causing his fatal illness, and was now suffering from its late consequences.

She wanted a lumbar puncture and when denied this presented herself to both the local A&E department and the sexually transmitted diseases (STD), clinic seeking this investigation. Refusing to see a psychiatrist, she did accept antidepressant medication and after three months her insistence on the cause of her ailments disappeared – although her physical symptoms did not.

Conclusions

Organic brain pathology and sensory impairment may confer vulnerability to psychosis, but other long-standing or ageing-related factors trigger the development of psychotic illness. Personality may determine how individuals respond to the last maturational task of life, the integration of the ego, with despair, fragmentation of the self, and the emergence of paranoid fears occurring in those who are unable to achieve this.[70] General practitioners working with older people who develop delusions, hallucinations, and hypochondriacal preoccupations therefore need to think about:

- the pre-morbid personality of the individual, using informant histories wherever possible to supplement their own knowledge and records
- any previous history of psychiatric disorder, particularly 'breakdowns' or prolonged hospital admissions in earlier life that might be signs of a psychotic episode or a major depressive illness
- current features suggestive of cognitive impairment, particularly loss of functional ability, or emotional lability, as well as memory loss
- other complaints suggesting a depressive disorder, especially anhedonia – the inability to find pleasure in anything – or multiple physical complaints
- visual and hearing impairments, which are often undetected or underestimated by both the patients and professionals.

Working up the patient with psychotic symptoms is very clearly a task for primary care professionals, but always with a view to referral and the involvement of other agencies. Treatment of psychosis in later life is complicated and requires specialist advice and multidisciplinary team input, even if referral is not always practical.

References

1 Sharma VK & Copeland JRM Presentation and assessment of depression in old age. In Ghose K (ed) *Antidepressants for elderly people.* Chapman & Hall, London 1989.

2 MacDonald AJD Do general practitioners miss depression in elderly patients? *British Medical Journal* 1986; **292**:1365–7.

3 Cooper B Psychiatric illness, epidemiology and the general practitioner. In Cooper B & Eastwood R (eds) *Primary health care and psychiatric epidemiology* Tavistock/Routledge, New York 1992.

4 Rabins PV Barriers to diagnosis and treatment of depression in elderly patients. *Am. J. Geriatr. Psych.* 1996; **4**:S79–S83.

5 Fogel BS & Fretwell M Reclassification of depression in the medically ill elderly. *Journal of the American Geriatricians Society* 1985; **33**:446–8.

6 La Vecchia C, Lucchini F, & Levi F Worldwide trends in suicide mortality, 1955–89. *Acta Psychologica Scandinavica* 1994; **90**:53–64.

7 Newmann JP Aging and depression. *Psychology and Ageing* 1989; **4**(2):150–65.

8 Gallo JJ, Rabins PV, & Iliffe S The 'research magnificent' in later life: psychiatric epidemiology and the primary health care of older adults *International Journal of Psychiatry in Medicine* 1997; **27**(3):185–204.

9 Iliffe s,Gould MM, Mitchley S, *et al.* Evaluation of brief screening instruments for depression, dementia and problem drinking in general practice. *British Journal of General Practice* 1994; **44**:503–7.

10 German PS, Shapiro S, Skinner EA, *et al.* Detection and management of mental health problems of older patients by primary care providers *Journal of the American Medical Association* 1987; **257**:489–93.

11 Girling DM, Huppert FA, Brayne C, *et al.* Depressive symptoms in the very elderly – their prevalence and significance. *International Journal of geriatric Psychiatry* 1995; **10**:497–504.

12 Flint AJ & Rifat SL Anxious depression in elderly patients: response to anti-depressant treatment. *American Journal of Geriatric Psychiatry* 1997; **5**:107–15.

13 Flint AJ & Rifat SL Two-year outcome of elderly patients with anxious depression. *Psychiat. Res.* 1997; **87**:11–13.

14 Exton Smith AN, Stanton BR, & Windsor ACM *Nutrition of housebound older people.* King Edward's Hospital Fund, London 1976.

15 Flint AJ Epidemiology and comorbidity of anxiety disorders in the elderly. *American Journal of Psychiatry* 1994; **151**:640–9.

16 Blanchard MR, Waterreus A, & Mann AH The nature of depression among older people in inner London, and their contact with primary care. *British Journal of Psychiatry* 1994; **164**:396–402.

17 Lindsay J, Briggs SK, & Murphy E The Guys/Age Concern survey prevalence rates

of cognitive impairment, depression and anxiety in an urban elderly community. *British Journal of Psychiatry* 1989; **155**:377–89.

18 Kramer M, German PS, Anthony JC, *et al.* Patterns of mental disorder among the elderly residents of Eastern Baltimore. *Journal of the American Geriatricians Society* 1985; **33**:236–45.

19 Beinfeld D Nosology and classification. In Copeland JRM, Abou-Saleh MT, & Blazer DG (eds) *Principles and practice of geriatric psychiatry.* John Wiley, Chichester 1994.

20 McWilliam C When to worry about anxiety. *Health & Ageing* 1998; **June:**47–50.

21 Katona CLE The epidemiology and natural history of depression in old age. In Ghose K (ed) *Antidepressants for elderly people.* Chapman & Hall, London 1989.

22 Beekman ATF, Kriegsman DMW, & Deeg DJH The association of physical health and depressive symptoms in the older population: age and sex differences. *Soc. Psychiatr. Psychiatr. Epidemiol.* 1995; **30**:32–8.

23 Kennedy GL, Kelman HR, & Thomas C The emergence of depressive symptoms in late life: the importance of declining health and increasing disability. *Journal of Community Health* 1990; **15**:93–104.

24 Evans S & Katona CLE The epidemiology of depressive symptoms in elderly primary care attenders. *Dementia* 1993; **4**:327–33.

25 Mofic HS & Paykel ES Depression in medical in-patients. *British Journal of Psychiatry* 1975; **126**:346–53.

26 Walker Z & Katona CLE Depression in elderly people with physical illness. In Robertson MM & Katona CLE (eds) *Depression and physical illness.* John Wiley, Chichester 1997.

27 Aromaa A, Raitasalo R, Reunanen K, *et al.* Depression and cardiovascular disease. *Acta Psychiatrica Scandinavica* 1994; **377**:77–82.

28 Ahern DK, Gorkin L, Anderson JL, *et al.* Biobehavioral variables and mortality or cardiac arrest. *American Journal of Cardiology* 1990; **66**:59–62.

29 Silverstone PH Depression increases mortality and morbidity in acute life-threatening medical illness. *J. Psychosom. Res.* 1990; **34**:651–7.

30 McQuellon RP & Reifler B Caring for the depressed elderly and their families. In Hughston GA, Christopherson VA, & Bonjean MJ (eds) *Aging & family therapy: practitioner perspectives on Golden Pond* Howarth, New York 1989.

31 Craig TKJ & Boardman AP Somatization in primary care settings in Bass E (ed) *Somatization: physical symptoms and psychological illness.* Blackwell Scientific Publications, Oxford 1990.

32 Craig TKJ & Boardman AP Somatization in primary care settings. In Bass C (ed) *Somatization: physical symptoms and psychological illness.* Blackwell Scientific Publications, Oxford 1990.

33 Conwell Y & Caine ED Rational suicide and the right to die: reality and myth. *New England Journal of Medicine* 1991; **325**:1100–3.

34 La Vecchia C, Lucchini F, & Levi F Worldwide trends in suicide mortality, 1955–1989. *Acta Psychiatrica Scandinavica.* 1994; **90**:53–64.

35 McIntosh J Older adults: the next suicide epidemic? *Suicide and Life-Threatening Behavior.* 1992; **22**:322–32.

36 Rutz W, Von Knorring L, & Walinder J Frequency of suicide on Gotland after systematic postgraduate education of general practitioners. *Acta Psychiatrica Scandinavica.* 1989; **80**:151–4.

37 Anon *Drugs & Therapeutics Bulletin* 1997; **35**(10):75–6

38 Rocca WA, Hofman A, Brayne C, *et al.* Frequency and distribution of Alzheimer's disease in Europe: a collaborative study of 1980–1990 prevalence findings. *Annals Neurology* 1991; **30**:381–90.

39 Hunter R, McGill L, Bosanquet N, *et al.* Alzheimer's disease in the United Kingdom: developing patient and carer support strategies to encourage care in the community. *Quality in Health Care* 1997; **6**:146–52.

40 Downs M The role of general practice and the primary care team in dementia diagnosis and management . *International Journal of Geriatric Psychiatry* 1996; **11**:937–42.

41 Iliffe S Can delays in the recognition of dementia in primary care be avoided? *Aging & Mental Health* 1997; **1**:7–10.

42 Haley WE, Clair JM, & Saulsberry K Family care-giver satisfaction with the medical care of their demented relatives. *Gerontologist* 1992; **32**:219–26.

43 Haug MR Elderly patients, care-givers and physicians: theory and practice on health care triads. *Journal of Health & Social Behaviour* 1994; **35**:1–12.

44 Alzheimer's Disease Society *Right from the start: primary health care and dementia.* Alzheimer's Disease Society, London 1995.

45 Towle A Changes in health care and continuing medical education for the 21st century. *British Medical Journal* 1998; **316**:301–4.

46 Rubin SM, Glasser ML & Werckle MA Examination of physicians' awareness of dementing disorders. *Journal of the American Geriatricians Society* 1987; **35**:1051–8.

47 Brodaty H, Howarth GC, Mant A, *et al.* General practice and dementia: a national survey of Australian GPs. *Medical Journal of Australia* 1994; **160**:10–14.

48 Wolff LE Do general practitioners and old-age psychiatrists differ in their attitudes to dementia? *International Journal of Geriatric Psychiatry* 1994; **10**:63–9.

49 Glosser G, Wexler D, & Balmelli M Physicians' and familes' perspectives on the medical management of dementia. *Journal of the American Geriatricians Society* 1985; **33**:383–91.

50 De Lepelaire JA, Heyrman J, Baro F, *et al.* How do general practitioners diagnose dementia? *Family Practice* 1994; **11**:148–52.

51 Morgan D & Zhao P the doctor–caregiver relationship: managing the care of family members with Alzheimer's disease. *Quality in health Res.* 1993; 3(2):133–64.

52 Haley W, Clair J, & Saulsberry K Family care-giver satisfaction with the medical care of their demented relatives. *Gerontologist* 1992; 32:219–26.

53 Chenoweth B & Spencer B Dementia: the experience of family care-givers. *Gerontologist* 1986; 26:267–72.

54 Eccles M, Clarke J, Livingstone M, *et al.* North of England Evidence-based Guidelines Development Project: summary version of evidence-based guidelines for the primary care management of dementia. *British Medical Journal* 1998; 317:802–8.

55 Kitwood T *Dementia reconsidered.* Open University Press , Milton Keynes 1997.

56 Kitwood T Towards a theory of dementia care: the interpersonal process. *Ageing & Society* 1993; 13:51–67.

57 Lacro JP, Harris MJ, & Jeste DV Late-life psychosis. in Murphy E & Alexopoulos G (eds) *Geriatric Psychiatry: key research topics for clinicians.* John Wiley, Chichester 1995.

58 Gurland BJ & Cross PS Epidemiology of psychopathology in old age. *Psychiatric Clinics of North America* 1982; 5(1):11–26.

59 McGlashlan TH Predictors of shorter-, medium,- and longer-term outcomes in schizophrenia. *American Journal of Psychiatry* 1986; 143:50–5.

60 Cohen CI Outcome of schizophrenia in later life: an overview. *Gerontologist* 1990; 30:790–7.

61 Harris MJ & Jeste DV Late-onset schizophrenia: an overview. *Schizophrenia Bulletin* 1988; 14:39–55.

62 Pearlson G & Rabins P The late-onset psychoses: possible risk factors. In Jeste DV & Sisook S (eds) *Psychiatric Clinics of North America*, vol. 11, pp. 33–46. WB Saunders, Philadelphia 1988.

63 Rockwell E, Krull AJ, Dimsdale J, *et al.* Late-onset psychosis with somatic delusions. *Psychsomatics* 1992; 35:66–72.

64 Gurian BS, Wexler D, & Baker EH Late-life paranoia: possible association with early trauma and infertility. *International Journal of Geriatric Psychiatry* 1992; 7:277–84.

65 Cooper JK, Mungas D, Verma M, *et al.* Psychotic symptoms in Alzheimer's disease. *International Journal of Geriatric Psychiatry* 1991; 6:721–6.

66 Berrios GE & Brook P Delusions and the psychopathology of the elderly with dementia. *Acta Psychiatrica Scandinavica* 1985; 72:296–301.

67 Jeste DV, Wragg RE, Salmon DP, *et al.* Cognitive deficits of Alzheimer disease patients with and without delusions. *American Journal of Psychiatry* 1992; 149:184–9.

68 Katona CLE *Depression in old age.* John Wiley, Chichester 1994.

69 Baldwin RC The nature, prevalence and frequency of depressive delusions. In Katona CLE & Levy R (eds) *Delusions and hallucinations in old age.* Gaskell, London 1992.

70 Hassett A The case for a psychological perspective on late-life psychosis. *Australian and New Zealand Journal of Psychiatry* 1997;31(1): 68–75.

CHAPTER TEN

Chronic obstructive pulmonary disease and asthma

Mr X. retired from his caretaker's job six years ago and moved to a new flat further up the hill from his general practitioner's surgery. Every month he would walk down to the surgery for a check on his lung function, his blood pressure (for he also had essential hypertension), and his weight. He had always been 'large', he said, but was mostly unconcerned about his obesity, (which gave him a BMI of 31), unless his clothes would not fit. The diagnosis of non-insulin-dependent diabetes mellitus (NIDDM) at 68 years came as no great shock to his GP, although it seemed to make Mr X. think very hard about what he ate, at least for a while. During the war and for the first part of his working life he had been a heavy smoker, never smoking less than one packet a day and sometimes two when he could afford to. He married late, and his only child was born when he was 43, at which point he gave up smoking instantly, after 26 years. His bronchitis became troublesome in his fifties, and every winter he had at least one course of antibiotics. He began to get wheezy after infections and became more and more breathless when he exerted himself. After his wife died suddenly from a stroke, when he was 63, he continued to struggle on foot to the supermarket every week, dropped into the pub once or twice a week, and travelled around his home city as much as he could by bus. An early convert to influenza immunization, he gratefully accepted the use of a salbutamol inhaler after a very alarming chest infection that precipitated an emergency admission to hospital, and added a steroid inhaler after a few months. During this admission the diagnosis of COPD was made after spirometry, but his GP continued to monitor his PEFR regularly. Although his PEFR measurements varied between 150 and 210 litres/min, it was difficult to see any pattern attributable to his medication, but Mr X. was sure that he was able to walk further and more quickly if he used the inhalers. Persistent ankle oedema and, latterly, some angina worsened his discomfort. The half-mile walk to the surgery was easy enough downhill, but the uphill return was a real struggle and he spent a lot of time resting on convenient walls. He died at the age of 72 following a myocardial infarction, whilst he was watching television.

The spectrum of respiratory diseases often overlaps with cardiovascular disease and deconditioning through prolonged lack of exercise to produce profound functional loss – the affected individual takes an hour to have a bath, struggles over short flights of stairs, and plans a walk of 100 yards to the corner newsagent as if it were a major expedition. Optimal treatment can improve the quality of life significantly, as it did for Mr X., yet respiratory diseases in later life are seemingly invisible, deprived of badges of disability like the zimmer frame or the unresponsive limbs of hemiparesis. Poorly covered in major texts about the health of older people compared with heart disease and stroke, they provoke little clinical enthusiasm and attract few services.

They are not trivial in their impact on people or populations. Bronchitis, emphysema, and asthma together cause long-standing illness in 8% of men and 5% of women aged 75 and over, a prevalence equivalent to those experiencing the consequences of non-fatal myocardial infarction, and twice that of stroke survivors.[1] Respiratory disorders, half of them being labelled bronchitis, make up 12% of GP consultations in the 75-and-over age group[2] but only 25% of people with COPD may be diagnosed,[3] partly because of the insidious onset of symptoms (cough, expectoration, and exercise intolerance). One in eight acute medical admissions may be due to COPD, and amongst older people admissions because of exacerbations of COPD are estimated as up to four times more frequent than admissions for angina.[4]

This burden of respiratory disease contributes to the high prevalence of disability in older age groups, constituting a major cause in 13% of disabled adults, comparable to mental health problems and disorders of the nervous system.[5] Mortality from respiratory disease rises with advancing age, being the cause of death of 9% of men and women aged 65–74, and of 20% of men and 16% of women aged 85 and over. Whilst this trend may reflect the choice of bronchopneumonia as an explanation of death on death certificates, the Medical Research Council also suggests that research into prevention of respiratory deaths in later life would be useful.[6]

Older people with COPD probably fare worse than those with asthma, where both diagnosis and treatment options are clearer. In the Central Manchester study[7] even the most severely disabled older patients with COPD received less support from statutory services than similarly disabled controls. In fact, their levels of support were similar to fit, age-matched controls. The disparity in service provision to this group was not explained by less potential exposure to multidisciplinary assessment, for the COPD group had the same rate of hospital admissions as those with other (non-respiratory) causes for their disabilities. The neglect of this category of patients may be inadvertent but it is pervasive across agencies, appearing in specialist and generalist care, in health services, and in social care as a form of therapeutic nihilism.

Towards better diagnosis

Part of the problem with COPD lies in the difficulty in making a diagnosis that guides action, with a tendency to merge respiratory diseases together (at least in later life) and treat them in the same way. Establishing a diagnosis can be important, even though there is an overlap in the clinical patterns of chronic respiratory diseases, because responses to therapeutic intervention may be very different.

A useful way to understand respiratory disease in later life is to see it as a group of overlapping disorders upon which progressive airways obstruction becomes superimposed. The component disorders can be defined as follows:

- COPD:
  - slowly progressive
  - characterized by airways obstruction that does not change markedly over months
  - may be accompanied by airways hyper-reactivity and partial reversibility
- chronic bronchitis:
  - cough with expectoration
  - for three of two successive years
  - not otherwise explicable
- emphysema:
  - permanent destructive enlargement of airways distal to terminal bronchiole, without fibrosis
- asthma:
  - inflammatory process
  - with expiratory airflow obstruction
  - reversible with inhaled or oral steroids.

Mr X. had COPD with some element of reversibility, but this was established during a hospital admission after spirometry, not by his GP who used a lung-function test more appropriate to asthma management. Distinguishing between asthma and COPD requires measurement of airways reversibility, using forced expiratory volume (FEV_1) as the measure rather than PEFR, which has implications for clinical practice. Peak flow measurement is of limited value because the airways collapse that can occur with COPD during forced manoeuvres means that PEFR does not necessarily distinguish between asthma and obstructive airways disease, cannot be used to stage severity and does not predict morbidity and mortality. On the other hand, (FEV_1) is:

- reproducible and standardizable
- comparable to normative data for age and sex
- diagnostic of airflow obstruction (see above)
- useful in estimating the reversibility of airflow obstruction helpful in staging the disease (see below)
- predictive of mortality (see below).

Assessing the severity of COPD is important for practitioners because it helps decision-making about referral for further investigation and pulmonary rehabilitation, and is a better guide to prognosis than symptoms or service use. Measurement of FEV_1 after nebulized bronchodilator therapy allows staging[8] as follows:

FEV$_1$ as percentage of predicted	Stage
60–79	Mild
40–59	Moderate
<40	Severe

Prognosis can be estimated from FEV$_1$ measurement, with very long survival times of 10 years or more for those with mild or moderate disease.[9]

Although the evidence base for producing clinical guidelines is weaker for COPD than for asthma,[10] we now have at least a pragmatic definition of COPD that can help practitioners: a chronic, slowly progressive disorder characterized by airways obstruction which does not change markedly over several months.[11] We could add to this a working definition as an FEV$_1$ less 70% of predicted and rising less than 15% after 5 mg of nebulized salbutamol.[7] The diagnosis and management of COPD can be summarized as in Figure 10.1.

Case management

Using these definitions to identify COPD cases allows us to target this group for interventions that are known to improve quality of life, increase self-esteem and social interaction, and reduce hospital admission rates.[12] The management plan is distinct from that of asthma, with the emphasis on:

- education
- smoking cessation
- use of bronchodilators even in the absence of demonstrable airways reversibility, if there is measurable functional benefit
- pragmatic use of inhaled corticosteroids
- promotion of physical activity
- use of long-term oxygen therapy
- immunization against influenza and pneumococcus.

Education

The insidious onset of symptoms and the slow decline in functional ability caused by COPD may be attributed to 'smoker's cough' and normal ageing, and patients with advanced disease may be unaware of what they have and why they are so disabled. There is an obvious argument for providing information to maximize patient self-efficacy (Box 10.1) and so improve morale, and there is evidence that a programme that combines education, tailored exercise, and systematic case management can improve exercise capability and quality of life in patients with moderate to severe COPD.[13] However, this requires input from a multidisciplinary team, immediately raising the issues of priorities, available resources, and skill mix for those commissioning and

Figure 10.1 The diagnosis and management of COPD (derived from the British Thoracic Society Guidelines, 1997).

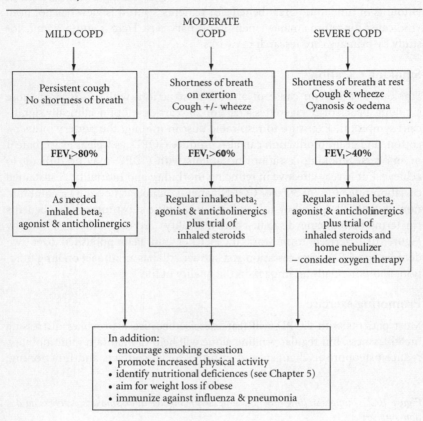

Box 10.1 *Patient information source*

The British Lung Foundation has produced and information leaflet on COPD for patients, based on the British Thoracic Society's guidelines. This is available from: The British Lung Foundation
                                    78 Hatton Gardens
                                    London EC1N 8 JR

providing services. Mr X. did not get this level of input, despite his GP's efforts to optimize case management, because in his area the local hospitals did not have a dedicated team with a systematic approach to COPD. So far the evidence of effectiveness of multidisciplinary interventions with COPD patients comes mainly from hospital outreach projects,[14] where admission is avoided or shortened, and from nurse-led projects that cross the interface between primary and secondary care.[15] Could the same approach be organized at PCG level, from within primary care, with the same effectiveness? GPs and practice nurses may take the view that labour-intensive, highly specialized educational work about the causes and consequences of COPD might consume large amounts of time to no great benefit for patients,[16] but this view has not been vindicated for asthma management in primary care. Here is another topic for study by primary care research networks.

Smoking cessation

Smoking is the main cause of airways obstruction, with 15–20% of those smoking a pack of 20 cigarettes a day for 20 years developing clinically significant symptoms. Exposure to respirable dust in mining, the pottery industry, cotton, and grain production can also produce COPD, as well as exacerbate it in smokers. Smoking cessation in patients with COPD may be difficult to achieve, but is very effective in reducing morbidity and mortality. A sustained cessation rate of up to 30% of COPD patients can be achieved by a combination of counselling, follow-up, and use of nicotine substitutes.[17] The benefits (in terms of reducing disability and mortality) are dramatic, as shown by Figure 10.2 derived from work by Fletcher and Peto published over two decades ago.[18] Smoking cessation at a late age still has an impact on lung function, and potentially an impact on the quality of life.

Promoting exercise

Most patients with COPD will fear exercise because it provokes distressing breathlessness, but regular walking alone will help to maintain joint mobility, reduce osteoporotic changes, and improve social contacts and functioning.

Figure 10.2 *Changes in lung function with advancing age in ex-smokers, smokers, and non-smokers*

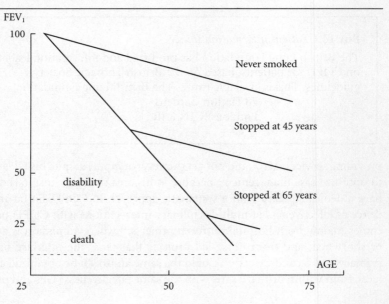

Mr X. kept walking as long as he could, probably preventing even greater weight gain and certainly maintaining his self-esteem and morale, but he might have done even better with more expert help. Aerobic exercise programmes improve functional ability in individuals with both asthma and COPD, but need to be supervised by an experienced therapist.[19] Primary care groups may want to consider whether there are sufficient trained physiotherapists or exercise therapists in their area to meet the needs of this patient population.

Medication use

Bronchodilators produce subjective rather than objective improvement in lung function, but this may be enough to improve exercise performance, perhaps by influencing mood in ways that were discussed in Chapter 5. About one in three patients with COPD will experience extra benefits from using higher doses of beta agonists by nebulizer,[20] although this has significant financial implications for both the patient and the health service.[21]

Inhaled or oral steroids can produce an improvement in both symptoms and FEV_1 in 10–15% of patients with apparent COPD, suggesting that they have a mixed pathology with some reversible component, and they may have a better five year survival if treated long term with inhaled steroids.[8] A trial of steroids is possible in the community, as shown in Box 10.2.

Box 10.2 *A trial of steroids in COPD*

Measure FEV_1 before and after, with twice-daily PEFR recordings at home.

Give steroids as either:

- oral prednisolone 30–40 mg daily for two weeks
- or inhaled beclamethasone 500 mcg twice daily for six weeks.

Significant reversibility is present if there is:

- an improvement in FEV_1 of >15% (equivalent to more than 200 ml)
- or an improvement in the mean PEFR between the first five days and the last five days of >20%.

Long-term oxygen therapy

Oxygen therapy is useful in reducing symptoms and improving function in patients with severe COPD who are persistently hypoxic when clinically stable, so should only be initiated after specialist assessment. Criteria for long-term oxygen therapy provision are:

- FEV_1 <1.5 litres and PaO2 <7.3 kPa

- or PaO_2 7.3–8.0 kPa and ankle oedema, hypercapnea, or nocturnal hypoxaemia
- after post-bronchodilator measurements on two occasions at least three weeks apart.

Long-term oxygen therapy should be used by non-smoking COPD patients for a minimum of 15 hours per day, at flow rates determined at assessment. There is an argument for intermittent oxygen use for symptom relief, especially when exertion produces marked oxygen desaturation, and such patients should also be assessed by specialists.

Immunization

Prevention of acute exacerbations of chronic respiratory disease by immunization against influenza reduces hospital admissions and mortality from acute respiratory illness,[22] with few adverse effects. The same appears to be true of immunization against pneumococcal pneumonia. Older people and those with heart disease, immunosuppression, other respiratory disease, and liver or renal failure, are particularly likely to develop pneumonia as a complication of influenza. Between 3000 and 4000 deaths are attributable to influenza each year, with 85% of them occurring in the 65-and-over age group, and a death rate 10 times higher can occur in epidemics. Influenza immunization has a powerful effect on these risks,[23] as shown in Table 10.1.

These figures may underestimate the beneficial impact of influenza immunization. A mathematical model based on an epidemiological study of the number of deaths that may have been avoided by influenza immunization amongst older people in France between 1980 and 1990[24] suggests that:

- many older people who die from influenza do not have their cause of death registered as such
- up to eight times as many deaths may be attributable to influenza than are registered
- the number of deaths avoided will vary dependent on vaccine effectiveness, but may be as many as 697 per 100 000 deaths.

Annual vaccination confers more protection than first-time immunization,

Table 10.1

Outcome measure	% cases prevented
Respiratory illness	49
Pneumonia	59
Hospital admission	56
Death	69

and systemic side-effects occur as often with influenza immunization as they do with placebo administration.[25]

Nevertheless there is still scepticism about the value of influenza immunization, amongst patients and professionals, and coverage of the at-risk population is still not complete, one study from general practice showing that only two-thirds of nursing and residential home occupants had been immunized, with no discernible relationship between immunization status and medical risk factors.[26] Public health physicians puzzle over the apparent lack of commitment amongst GPs to immunize against influenza, and amongst at-risk patients to take up the offer of immunization, but it does not take much experience of primary care to understand why immunization is not complete. Leaving aside the issues about how much value is attached to older people discussed in Chapter 2, there are two important clinical considerations: the mortality rate is low, even on the most favourable interpretation of data (see above), and there are many other causes of lower respiratory tract infections in older people that are clinically indistinguishable from influenza.

If the number of deaths avoided by influenza vaccination is as high as 697 per 100 000, as the French model suggests it could be, few GPs will notice the lives saved – seven out of every 1000 *deaths*. This is not the same as the visible reduction in the number of strokes, or admissions with acute asthma, experienced over a decade or so of professional work, and does not provide the same positive feedback on professional activity. Other clinical conditions also produce a burden of respiratory illness that translates into tangible workload. For example, respiratory syncitial viruses (RSV) may cause about the same number of emergency admissions of older people to hospital with chest infections.[27] Effective immunization against influenza may more than halve the admissions due to influenzal pneumonia, but only reduce the viral pneumonia workload by a quarter. This reduction in caseload might be apparent to hospital doctors, but not necessarily to the admitting general practitioners. Add to this the impact of rhinovirus infections in older people, which outnumber influenza A sixfold and which produce prolonged lower respiratory tract symptoms in two-thirds of those infected,[28] and the influenza picture becomes very unclear for practitioners. Influenza vaccination would have to be very effective to make an impact on this burden of morbidity and the workload that it generates. Perhaps we should be surprised how many older people are immunized against influenza, not how many are not. Paradoxically, the large numbers of older people in the community who receive antibiotics for their prolonged lower respiratory symptoms may inadvertently be contributing to the growth in antibiotic resistance in pneumococcus[29] which makes immunization against this bacterial infection increasingly necessary.

This management package may be one that primary care teams may wish to develop in conjunction with specialist services, but there are significant implications for training in primary care and service provision at specialist level. The management of asthma in younger age groups has been taken up in primary care as a core function, but by comparison with COPD management is relatively simple. We have much to learn about COPD, both at a personal and professional level and in terms of its prevention, natural history, and susceptibility to medical intervention. Respiratory specialists may have an important educational role as well as offering specific clinical functions, including:

- diagnostic support
- strategies for optimizing treatment
- assessment for long-term oxygen therapy
- pulmonary rehabilitation programmes, including exercise promotion, dietary advice, and patient education.

As we have shown, diagnosis of COPD is relatively straightforward once FEV1 is used as the measure of lung function, but clinical symptoms may be misleading and other conditions can complicate the picture. For example, a patient with apparent severe COPD, chest hyperinflation, and diminished breath sounds may have cor pulmonale with:

- peripheral oedema and cyanosis
- raised jugular venous pressure (JVP)
- congestive hepatomegaly
- a cardiac murmur (pulmonary/tricuspid regurgitation).

Making the distinction is important in clinical management, and primary care workers taking on themselves the job of managing COPD in the community will need to be aware of such potential confounding diagnoses in an older population with multiple pathology. Mr X. had COPD, hypertension, and NIDDM, and he finally died from ischaemic heart disease, not his respiratory pathology, but he had peripheral oedema from another cause and might have been mistakenly diagnosed during an episode of acute breathlessness as being in ventricular failure. Specialist assessment, albeit triggered by an acute admission rather than by referral, provided him with a diagnosis and the right approach to treatment, but it did not offer a fuller package of pulmonary rehabilitation services. Pulmonary rehabilitation may be very effective, but most PCGs will not yet have access to well-established multidisciplinary teams of respiratory physicians, nurse practitioners, dieticians, and physiotherapists.

Asthma

We will end with a discussion of asthma, which when chronic can be mistaken for COPD as easily as vice versa, and when acute can be difficult to distinguish from heart failure. Diagnosis in the acute setting may be problematic, the signs of acute asthma and pulmonary oedema being similar in many instances, so that the distinguishing features may be presence of diuretics or inhalers at the patient's bedside. Emergency treatment is similar, and given the life-threatening nature of both conditions, should be instigated before diagnostic certainty is achieved.

Chronic asthma is easier to see if the diagnostic processes described earlier in this chapter are followed, and also to treat because management guidelines have a more robust evidence base than they do for COPD. GPs and practice nurses are now likely to know the British Thoracic Society guidelines on asthma management[30] in great detail, thanks to sustained educational efforts over recent years, and we are not going to repeat any more than their most basic themes.

The severity of asthma determines which step of a treatment ladder each patient occupies, and relies on objective measurement more than subjective symptoms. Whilst FEV_1 measurement (after bronchodilator use) may be essential to make the diagnosis of asthma, routine monitoring can be done using PEFR measurements. The treatment steps are:

(1) occasional use of relief bronchodilators
(2) regular inhaled anti-inflammatory agents
(3) high-dose inhaled steroids or low-dose inhaled steroids plus inhaled long-acting beta-agonist bronchodilators
(4) high-dose inhaled steroids and regular bronchodilators
(5) addition of oral steroids.

There is little reason to think that patient education and involvement in home monitoring and modifying treatment regimes where necessary is any less important for older patients than for younger ones, but there may be important cohort differences in knowledge and expectations that need inves-tigation and clarification. The apparent diminished perception of airways narrowing in later life makes reliance on subjective symptoms even more unreliable than in younger patients, so PEFR monitoring is important. The selection of the best inhaler device is also important, with some evidence that older people benefit from using large-volume spacer devices. All of these activities – understanding written management plans, monitoring lung func-tion at home, adjustment of treatment – may be compromised by cognitive impairment or depression, and require involvement of family members by the primary care team. Asthma is a good example of how primary care for older people takes the practitioner out of the one-to-one contact in the consulting room into a wider world of teamwork and public involvement in solving clinical problems. We will now return to these themes to describe options for primary care development in the next decade that will benefit an ageing population.

Key points

For practitioners:

- Every practice should have a spirometer, and both GPs and practice nurses should know how to use it and how to interpret the results.
- An industrial and occupational history can be important in understand-ing the origins of COPD, and may have medico-legal implications
- Information about the causes and consequences of COPD may have an important impact on the effectiveness of clinical management.

- Immunization against influenza and pneumococcal pneumonia are effective in reducing mortality and morbidity, and present coverage of the most vulnerable older people can be improved.
- Tailored management plans for asthma management in older patients should be as routine as they are in younger cohorts.

For clinical governance and commissioning in PCGs:

- Training programmes for COPD recognition and management in primary care are needed, perhaps on a scale to match those for asthma.
- Pulmonary rehabilitation is effective, but is under-resourced.

For primary care research networks:

- The best approaches to smoking cessation in older COPD patients need further study, with motivational interviewing a promising technique.
- Exercise promotion as a therapy for older people needs further investigation to find the best way to incorporate it into everyday practice.

References

1 Office of Population Census and Surveys, Social Survey Division *General Household Survey 1988* HMSO, London 1990.

2 Wilkin D and Williams EI Patterns of care for the elderly in general practice. *Journal of the Royal College of General Practitioners* 1986; **36**:567–70.

3 Manfreda J, Mas Y, & Litven W Morbidity and mortality from COPD. *American Journal of Respiratory Disease* 1989; **140**:S19–S26.

4 McCormick A, Fleming D, & Chalton J *Morbidity statistics from general practice: fourth national study 1991–92* OPCS, London 1995.

5 Martin J, Meltzer H, & Elliot D *The prevalence of disability amongst adults.* OPCS, HMSO, London 1988.

6 Medical Research Council *The health of the UK's elderly people.* MRC, London 1994.

7 Yohannes AM, Roomi J, & Connolly MJ Elderly people at home disabled by chronic obstructive pulmonary disease. *Age & Ageing* 1998; **27**(4):523–5.

8 Raasheed M & Allen MB COPD: clinical features and diagnosis. *Geriatric Medicine* 1998; **28**(1):31–33.

9 Traver GA, Clive MG, & Burrows B Predictors of mortality in COPD. *American Review of Respiratory Disease* 1979; **119**:895.

10 Taylor DR Chronic obstructive pulmonary disease. *British Medical Journal* 1998; **316**:1475.

11 British Thoracic Society Standards of Care Committee Guidelines for the management of chronic obstructive pulmonary disease. *Thorax* 1997; **52**(5).

12 Miles-Tapping C Home care for chronic obstructive pulmonary disease: impact of the Iqualit programme. *Arch. Med. Resp.* 1994; **55**:163–75.

13 Lacasse Y, Wong E, & King D Meta-analysis of respiratory rehabilitation in COPD. *Lancet* 1996; **348**:1115–9.

14 Gravil JH, Al-Rawas OA, Cotton MM, *et al.* Home treatment of exacerbations of chronic obstructive pulmonary disease by an acute respiratory assessment service. *Lancet* 1998; **351**:1853–5.

15 Callaghan S The RITE stuff. *Nursing Times* 1998; **94**(49):42–3.

16 Pearson M COPD rehabilitation. *Geriatric Medicine* 1997; **27**(4):53–5.

17 Anthonisen NR, Connet JE, & Kiley JP Effects of smoking intervention and the use of inhaled anti-cholinergic bronchodilator on the rate of decline of FEV1. The Lung Health Study. *Journal of the American Medical Association* 1994; **272**:1497–505.

18 Fletcher C & Peto R The natural history of chronic airflow limitation. *British Medical Journal* 1977; **1**:1645–8.

19 Young A & Dinan S Fitness for older people. *British Medical Journal* 1994; **309**:331–4.

20 Raashed M & Allen MB COPD: guidelines for management. *Geriatric Medicine* 1998; **28**(2):57–9.

21 Dowson L & Allen M Nebulisers: applications and limitations of therapy. *Geriatric Medicine* 1998; **28**(4).

22 NHS Centre for Reviews & Dissemination Influenza vaccination and older people. *Effectiveness Bulletin* 1996; **2**:1.

23 Gross PA, Hermogenes AW, Sacks HS, *et al.* The efficacy of influenza vaccine in elderly persons: a meta-analysis and review of the literature. *Annals of International Medicine* 1995;123:519-527

24 Carrat F & Valleron AJ Influenza mortality among the elderly in France, 1980–1990: how many deaths may have been avoided through vaccination? *Journal of Epidemiology & Community Health* 1995; **49**:419–25.

25 Govaert TME, Aretz K, & Masurel N Adverse reactions to influenza vaccine in elderly people. *British Medical Journal* 1993; **302**:988–90.

26 Evans MR & Wilkinson EJ How complete is immunisation coverage? A study in 75 nursing and residential homes for elderly people. *British Journal of General Practice* 1995; **45**:419–21.

27 Falsey AR, Cunningham CK, & Barker WH Respiratory syncitial virus and influenza A infections in the hospitalised elderly. *Journal of Infectious Diseases* 1995; **172**:389–94.

28 Nicholson KG, Kent J, Hammersley V, *et al.* Risk factors for lower respiratory complications of rhinovirus infections in elderly people living in the community: prospective cohort study. *British Medical Journal* 1996; **313**:1119–23.

29 Tomasz A The pneumococcus at the gates. *New England Journal of Medicine* 1995; **333**:514–5.

30 British Thoracic Society Guidelines on asthma management 1995: review and position statement. *Thorax* 1997; **52**(1):S1–S21.

CHAPTER ELEVEN

Developing primary care services for older people

In this final section of the book we return to, and expand upon, the earlier themes explored in the first four chapters. We examine the potential for improvement and change in services for older people by considering issues which focus beyond the care of *an* individual and beyond the activities of *an* individual primary care professional. This chapter includes a discussion of:

- proactive work with older people
- identifying issues for action in primary care
- local voices influencing change
- resource and service mapping
- methods of analysis and prioritization of new developments.

Most primary care practitioners experience their work as dealing with the individual person – whether as a consultation or a referral because that is how the 'work' arrives. During the nineties primary care professionals have experienced major service changes imposed from without through legislative and fiscal changes, the possible exception to this imposition being fundholding, which was not only voluntary but also inspired some practices to think in innovative ways. Most notably this external imposition included the introduction of:

- the general practitioner contract in 1990
- the 'internal market' in local authorities and health authorities
- the community care reforms
- and national efficiency measures in local authority and health service budgets.

Many of these developments were predicated on an understanding of population or service design and gave impetus for the development of information and business systems which supported that perspective, e.g. practice population targets in health promotion; annual business plans for community health services . The introduction of primary care groups with a responsibility for implementing local health improvement plans (HImPs)[1] which link to the local authority-led joint improvement Plans (JIPs)[2] for vulnerable people strengthens the opportunities to examine and develop services for older people as a population in a particular area. Between the individual (the micro level) and the area population – health authority or local authority defined – (the macro level), there is the intermediate level of a practice, locality, and primary care group populations (the meso level). It is at this level that there is most scope for the development activities which will make population planning and developments (at the macro level) more effective. We argue that in order to become more proactive, rather than reactive, in the service development for older people, the culture of primary care professionals and services needs to incorporate the following elements more significantly than at present:

- value working with older people and an ageing population
- a shift from just responding to individuals to a wider population focus
- working in closer partnership with patients and carers
- collaboratively work with the voluntary sector and statutory social care
- a whole-system view of care, not just a partial view of a section of it
- an increase in the knowledge base about how to make change happen and how to evaluate it.

Becoming proactive in working with older people

In the discussion about case management, and the subsequent clinical chapters, we have argued for the adoption of a systematic process to identify the action that needs to be made for individuals and whole groups, involving different perceptions in that process. The potential for the symbiosis between practices and PCGs is there but as yet unclear . The principles of this systematic process must include:

(1) identification through needs assessment methods of the health and health care problems of older people
(2) identification of the statutory voluntary services and community resources available to older people
(3) prioritization of the problems identified through step 1 using clear criteria
(4) development of plans to address prioritized problems (3), in collaboration with other disciplines and agencies (identified in step 2) with a knowledge of the range of options
(5) implementation of the plans so developed
(6) their evaluation and review before returning to the development cycle.

During the nineties a number of systematic processes gained ground in primary health care which address elements of this process, e.g. clinical audit, caseload/workload profiling in community nursing, locality commissioning. and business planning cycles. The creation of quasi-internal markets in the public sector during the nineties has given groups of primary health care professionals very different types of experiences of systematic processes. The experiences of fundholding (as individual practices or as part of consortia) exposed more GPs than ever before to the issues of systematic service review, although not necessarily reviews of their own services. Community nurses, professionals allied to medicine, and social workers are more likely to have experienced an entire service review by commissioners or outside agencies.

In addition, two systematic processes containing many of the principles outlined above have been explored within primary care. These are the use of total quality management principles[3] and the use of community-orientated primary care (COPC) methods.[4] TQM principles rely on a dynamic system whereby the processes of care are systematically reviewed from the patients' and professionals' perspective to form the basis for strategies for improvement and development.[5] Emphasis is given to the idea that services are used internally in the organization as well as externally and the needs of both these groups of users must be assessed. COPC principles offer a framework in which to develop strategies for service change based on prioritization informed by patient and local community views.[6] Stages include a community diagnosis, prioritization of the issues to be addressed, more detailed analysis of the problems followed by plans to address it, then implementation and finally evaluation.

We will return to the key lessons from these explorations and experiences of the nineties as we discuss elements of this systematic approach.

Identifying issues for action

At the practice level, a systematic process needs the sponsorship, support, and commitment from the partners and the practice team. Chapter 4 described the need to have clear team aims and objectives. In placing a clear objective, e.g. 'to review the current provision of health care for older people and identify aspects for service development and improvement', in the practice plan for the year and agreeing that with the wider team, the first step has been taken in conferring status on the project and value on the health care needs of older people. Likewise the inclusion of a similar objective within the primary care development plan by a PCG will signal the importance of the issue, and also commits the PCG to action and subsequent review . To turn this objective into action will need decisions on who does what and when, and no objectives should be set without such decisions. Many commentators identify the futility and frustration of undertaking initial review or health needs assessment when there is no prior commitment to action on the basis of the findings.[7]

The first step for any primary health care team must be to define what questions it wants to answer . In the widest sense the team will want to ask:

- What are we doing for the older people in our practice?
- What is the health and illness profile of our older people like?
- How well are we doing for the older people in this practice?
- What should we be doing better?

This mix of questions has been deliberate to reflect the need to be realistic about the nature of service development and the variety of information required. We are going to use the term 'health needs assessment' to describe this starting point.

At the outset there needs to be clarity that needs assessment involves three distinct stages which help point the way to an agenda for action:

(1) description
(2) analysis
(3) prioritization.

The concept of need is complex and in relation to health often complicated by different professional perspectives. Bradshaw[8] provided a taxonomy of four types of needs, based on the criteria from which they were derived:

(1) *felt needs* as perceived by the individual
(2) *expressed needs* as the *felt need* turned into action or demand
(3) *normative needs* as those defined by professionals or experts according to prescribed standards or practices
(4) *comparative needs* as those identified by comparison with others in similar situations/locations/conditions.

This categorization illuminates both the relative nature of the concept and the source of potential conflicts in assessing need (Box 11.1). There is much evidence that professional and consumer perspectives on need and priorities differ.[9] A recent survey of practices in the North of England identified that practitioners perceived one barrier to undertaking population-based assessment of need was that patient-expressed need would not necessarily equate with 'real' need.[10] Another source of tension is that of the definition of health needs. While the health service has defined health need in terms of the population's ability to benefit from health care services,[11] the determinants of ill health and the solutions are often beyond the boundaries of the health service.

Box 11.1 *The different perspectives on the concept of need.*

Self-perceived needs (felt need) depends on knowledge of my situation and health. For this to become an *expressed need* I need to have knowledge of what health and social care might be able to offer me and value the cost of doing something about it as worthwhile. In this my perception may not conform with the professional's perception of need – *normative need* (eg. consultation with the GP for a minor cold). Professionals may perceive a need (*normative*) which I and others in my situation (*felt need*) do not perceive as a need, for example the need for smoking cessation advice or compulsory detainment for psychiatric care.

These issues help in understanding the interplay between the three main approaches to needs assessment:

(1) the epidemiological (focused on estimates of prevalence and incidence)
(2) the comparative (using standardized measures such as mortality ratios or deprivation measures such as the Jarman underprivileged area score)
(3) the community/user defined (using patient and local resident perceptions of their priorities).

The purpose of assessment is to identify options for action. In order to identify problems and issues, information must be available on how (and to what extent) needs are currently met. Stevens and Sadler[12] have described how epidemiological-based needs assessment has moved from the scientific, quantitative concerns of prevalence and incidence to incorporate knowledge of effectiveness of interventions as well as knowledge of current services.

Within primary and community care there is a long history of examples which use the three approaches to health needs assessment (epidemiological, comparative, and informed by the local users) to acknowledge the multi-factorial causation of ill health. 'Community-orientated general practice'[13] is the term that has been used often in the medical literature while health visiting, social and community work have used the terms 'community profiling or health profiling'[14,15] Primary care professionals have also been involved in this type of needs assessment as part of wider health promotion activities, such as the Health Cities movement[16] based on the principles of the World Health Organization strategy *Health for All by the Year 2000*, and community development initiatives.[17]

So what are the experiences of primary care professionals involved in needs assessment? One major lesson from all the literature on health needs assessment in primary care is that it is a process which takes time and a range of expertise.[18,19] There seem to be three ways this has been addressed:

1. Additional resources have been identified to undertake the task – often as an experiment or pilot. In these examples the finance has been translated into additional public health (community) nurse time,[20,21] or sessions from public health registrars[22] attached to the primary care team, or additional general practitioner time.[23]
2. The primary care team has worked collaboratively with others locally to undertaken the task.[24] These inevitably move beyond one practice population and focus on neighbourhoods and localities.
3. There has been a wider initiative to produce information aggregated at practice population/service level to feed into or kickstart the process. Many health authorities provide comparative practice profiles using key practice data[25] while in other areas a system of using the skills of practice- based nurses and health visitors have been used in elaborating these profiles.[26]

Common problems have been identified in all these experiences about the accessibility and relevance of information collected in primary health care services. Without fail, practices and primary care professionals trying to undertake this work have found that:

- There has been a deficit between their current information collection (manual and electronic) and its relevance to a systematic needs and service assessment. As the National Information Strategy has pointed out, much data collection has been an administrative task rather than an attempt to capture relevant health, health care, and outcome information.
- There is a gulf between health and local authority information on service utilization.
- Useful information systems with accurate data entry are only developed when the primary care team members start actively using the information to plan and develop services.
- Most of the available demographic and epidemiological information is based on wards and enumeration areas which may be served by any number of general practices. Trying to use this data to inform practice population needs assessment is problematic.

The many developments in information technology based in general practice have begun to point ways forward on the first two issues,[27] while innovative systems are being tested which link social service and community health data.[28] Although the lack of co-terminosity of different agencies' boundaries remains a problem for individual practices, it is not necessarily so for PCGs with their locality focus. Reconciling the information needs of the PCG and the individual practice will inevitably become a major issue as PCGs move forward with their agendas of primary care service development and clinical governance.

Local voices

Another common problem in undertaking health needs assessment has been the challenge of engaging local user and community perspectives into the process. Many of the general practice and community health services' needs assessment processes have been unable to incorporate this perspective. At the same time there is an increasingly powerful lobby for incorporating user views, particularly in local authorities where there is a strong culture and tradition to support it. The change of culture in the health service is happening but reflects the idiosyncratic nature of provision, particularly in primary care. Barriers to this cultural change include fears of being inundated by demands which cannot be meet as well as a belief that the patients' perspectives may not be valuable . More than that, the ability of how to assist patients (and particularly older people) to engage with needs and service assessment processes is not well developed. Many commentators are critical of satisfaction surveys which become self-fulfilling prophecies, influenced by issues such as the intimate relationship between, and dependency of, some older peoples on their doctors and nurses.[29]

However, there are a range of sources and methods for gathering user perspectives, including:

- information from complaints and appreciation procedures for the practice, community, and local authority staff

- suggestion boxes in practices, health centres, and other relevant sites
- surveys and questionnaires of service users – either specifically concerned with patient satisfaction or added to specific audit packages such as District Nurse Monitor.[30] Both quantitative and qualitative approaches have been used in these
- views from patient participation groups[31] established to provide patient perspectives on the health and health care services
- specific panels or groups of service users for consultation
- information from the locality (rather than the practice population) through community development projects using a range of methods, including rapid participatory appraisal[32] and profiling.[33]

Box 11.2 provides some sources of information on these methods relevant to primary care. User input presents many challenges both to service users and to the professionals. In some instances these have been overcome by bringing expertise in to the primary care team to undertake some of this work. Primary care teams have used facilitators from organizations such as the College of Health,[34] others have employed or linked with community development workers.[35] Very few publications focus on specific issues of how to involve older users with a spectrum of experiences. including those who are frail or housebound, those who act as advocates and interpreters for other older people, and those who actively provide care to other older people (including volunteer organizations or good neighbours).[36] Proactive consultation with older people in these groups requires the consideration of practical support (for example provision of 'relative sitting' or T-loop induction systems in premises) as well as innovative methods such as telephone conference discussions. One strong message from those writing about their experiences is that in order to demonstrate the value placed on older people's views, acknowledgement and action needs to follow consultation.

Box 11.2 *Resource information on including user views*

- National Consumer Council *In partnership with patients: Involving the community in general practice.* Handbook for GPs and practice staff, NCC London 1995.
- Thornton P & Tozer R *Involving older people in planning and evaluating community care: a review of initiatives.* Social Policy Research Unit, University of York 1994.
- Pritchard P *Involving patients in general practice: a practical guide.* Royal College of General Practice, London 1993.
- McIver S *Information on obtaining the views of users of pri mary health care services: consumer feedback resource.* King's Fund, London 1991.
- Joule N *Choices and opportunities for user involvement in the primary care-led NHS.* Greater London Association of Community Health Councils 1995.

The following three case examples show some different methods of consultation with older people. They serve to illustrate the increasing body of knowledge available to guide this work and the nature of the different outputs of value at this 'meso' planning level.

Case example 1 – Views on health services for older people in Kensington, Chelsea, and Westminster, London.
Kensington and Chelsea Community Health Council ran separate focus group interviews of GPs and older people (who were users of 15 different community groups) to talk about their perceptions of issues in health care for older people that needed addressing. The groups were asked to identify aspects of services that were good and should be replicated elsewhere and aspects of services that required improvement. The GPs and the older people held a number of views in common on the areas that needed improvement including:

- difficult physical access to many premises
- problems in transport to attend health service appointments
- lack of information on how to access health and community services
- the shortage of physiotherapy and chiropody services
- premature discharge of older people from hospital.

There were a number of areas that only one group or other identified issues of concern. The report made a series of recommendations to the health authority and commissioners as well as feeding back the results to the participants.

Kensington, Chelsea and Westminster Community Health Council, *GP Services and Older People.* Kensington, Chealsea and Westminster Community Health Council, London 1997.

Case example 2 – Community-led assessment of health needs of older people: Perceptions of Older people in Knightswood, Glasgow – health survey.
Survey methods were used by a group of local volunteers (the Knightswood Health Forum) working in community premises to investigate older people's perceptions of their health and health concerns .

One of the most serious concerns raised in the survey was the difficulty the older people had in heating their homes and the effects this had on their health. The survey found a strong relationship between how often people felt sad or depressed and the problems they experienced in keeping their homes warm. On this issue the Knightswood Health Forum planned to (i) investigate the issue further, (ii)seek ways to increase information and services available to older people to maximize heat in the home, and (iii) explore ways of increasing benefit and allowance uptake linked to other services in the area, e.g. GP surgeries.

Chaplin J Material and Social Poverty in Old Age: Knightswood Health Forum provides an Agenda for Action. *Community Health Action* 1997; **43**:8.

Case example 3 – Assessing community care needs within general practice in Liverpool
Surveys were undertaken by a practice team using an additional member of staff to determine the needs and sufficiency of service provision to practice patients over 75 and those likely to come within the framework of the community care legislation. Postal questionnaires were used as well as interviews to those with

mental health problems. Data was organized into four areas:

- people at risk
- services used
- current needs for services
- gaps in service provision.
  Outcomes included:
- areas for the Primary health care team to focus on in the future, including developing 'in house' methods of assessment of people with complex care needs, creating a proactive central point of access and contact
- detailed resource pack of local services
- improved links with other services through the referrals and meetings to learn of services.

Lloyd Jones H and Dorwick C Assessing community care needs within general practice. *Health and social care in the Community* 1996; **4(4)**: 234–5.

Resource and service mapping

The use of this element is more than just listing local services/resources, but describing to what degree older people are able to access them and how they are used. In many instances this part of the process has an immediate impact for a team as it provides a form of networking, often exposing some members of the team to services that they either never knew of or did not actively appreciate how that resource could be of use to older people.[37]

Table 11.1 provides an outline version of the data, the rationale, and the potential source in a health needs assessment process focused on older people in practice populations . This type of preplanning is essential before embarking on any data collection; fundamentally there has to be answer to why do you want the data and what are you going to do with the data when you get it? A number of commentators have questioned the value of undertaking needs assessment work at the practice population level[38] or placing too much reliance on the data generated from general practice and community health services.[39] However, to believe there is only value on undertaking all this work at PCG level is to ignore the need for practice ownership and collaboration if services are to develop at the primary care team level, an issue that is developed further in Chapter 12 . All primary care teams need to be able to answer the question 'how well are we doing for the older people for whom we are responsible?' The real potential for improvement of primary care for older people lies in apportioning some elements of the needs assessment process to the primary care team and other parts to the PCG. Each party then feeds the other with information so there is a creative symbiosis.

Analysis and prioritization

Judgements on data are based on values and priorities. In undertaking any health needs assessment these are often implicit rather than explicit. The analysis is trying to understand the significance of the data, invariably in terms of comparisons. A needs assessment methodology which draws on the

Table 11.1 *An outline template for the health needs assessment of a population of older adults*

Data	Source of data	Rationale for data	Sources of comparative data
1. Demographic data			
Demographic data of the people registered with the practice aged over 65 and over 75, including:	• Practice computerized patient lists	• Understanding of the volume of people in these age groups as a denominator	• Health authority data on other practice populations
• number and percentage of the practice population • gender • ethnicity • living alone • marital/cohabitation status • in receipt of state income support/housing benefit • caring for another frail or dependent other person in the home • caring for a significant other person in an institutional setting • housebound • nursing and residential home residents	• Age/sex registers • Annual over-75 screening activities records	• Identification of the extent of factors which may significantly affect individual older people's health and the workload of the primary care team	• Ward and enumeration district census data from the local public health department • Local authority reports related to their responsibilities in social services, leisure, housing, and education • Voluntary sector organizations' surveys

Table 11.1 Continued

Data	Source of data	Rationale for data	Sources of comparative data
2. Mortality data			
Numbers of deaths by cause and venue (i.e. home or hospital) over the preceding five years for people in these two age groups	• Practice mortality and bereavement register	• Identification of the volume of, and types of, terminal care needs within the population	• Age-specific mortality rates by ward and small area from the public health department
3. Morbidity data			
Numbers, percentage, and incidence of people in these age groups with: • hypertension • cardiovascular accident • diabetes • asthma • COPD • incontinence by type • dementia by stage • depression • sensory problems • leg ulcers • carcinoma by type	• Practice computerized patient lists • Chronic disease registers • Annual over-75 screening activities	• Identification of the volume and significant health problems experienced by this population and the consequent skills and knowledge requirements of those providing care • Identification of potential aspects of ill health which are not being identified as systematically as expected	• Age-specific in patient episodes by morbidity ward and small area from the public health department • Incidence data from other practices captured in baseline audits with the local MAAG or similar sources • Population prevalence and incidence estimates in national reports of Royal Colleges, groups, task forces, etc. and other authoritative sources

- alcohol dependency
- fractured bones in the past year
- accidents in the past year
- people with three or more of the above conditions
- concerns of neglect or abuse

4. Access to and utilization of service

- Use and frequency of consultation with GP, practice nurse, district nurse, specialist services, and professionals allied to medicine by relevant morbidity group
- Patients with a community care assessment and receiving services
- Carers with a community-care carers' needs assessment
- Use of local authority-funded services such as home carers, orange disabled parking badge

- Practice computerized data
- Data from district nurse/community health service activity collection processes
- Social services-held data

- Identification of level of multidisciplinary activity
- Identification of level of access to, and use of, primary care services

- Nationally available data, e.g. Morbidity Statistics from General Practice,[40] Health and Lifestyle Studies [41,42]
- General Household Survey, local authority and health authority

Table 11.1 *Continued*

Data	Source of data	Rationale for data	Sources of comparative data
5. Clinical and service effectiveness			
• Information that provided an assessment of activities of the professional or services against intentions or criteria	• Significant event reports • Audit studies • Service reviews • Evaluation studies	• Identification of current developmental work • Identification of services' aspects currently being developed	As column 2, and national
6. Perceptions of health needs and issues			
• Patients • Carers • Professional • Administrative/support staff and ancillary staff	• Team (staff) meetings' minutes • Group discussions with local older people • Patient participation groups' surveys • Suggestion boxes	• Identification of issues not visible through statistics • Identification of issues from the different experiences of receiving and providing health care	• Local reports from voluntary and statutory services • National patient survey

7. Local community resources for older people

Mapping local resources/ services/self-help groups for older people (including non-age specific) relevant to:
- promoting health of older people
- maintenance of health
- maintenance of indepence
- providing care

- Local service resource index provided by library services, local authority, voluntary group
- Service/resource guides from local authority and voluntary sector
- Team members adding local knowledge

- To provide the 'whole' picture of the resources available locally beyond the primary care team
- Other service/resource mapping in areas of similar geographics or geographical features

approaches outlined in Table 11.1 will use comparisons from a range of local and national information, including:

- demographic ratios
- prevalence/incidence
- service availability
- service use/access
- provision of service to population and weighted population ratios
- user views
- clinical guidance and protocols, both locally devised and those endorsed through the National Institute for Clinical Effectiveness (NICE)
- service standards and specifications detailed in previous contracts and now in service specifications and financial frameworks (SSAFF)[43]
- new national framework specifying services' standards and provision for older people.[44]
- quality indicators.

Analysis must focus on the questions the needs assessment sets out to answer. The objective may be to identify deficits in the process and outcome of health and social care, or it may be to understand more clearly the antecedents of the health deficits. In order to move from this stage to a plan for action, the identified issues have to be prioritized. This element is rarely made explicit in the accounts of needs assessment in primary care.

Community-orientated primary care is unusual in that it provides a framework for prioritizing issues[45] identified through a community diagnosis (needs assessment process). This framework uses a scoring system for each of the following criteria:

- size of the problem (prevalence/incidence)
- severity of problems in their effect on morbidity and mortality
- availability of effective intervention
- acceptability/feasibility of the interventions to users and the team
- community involvement
- costs and resources.

While this looks a logical, impartial way forward, the descriptions of the COPC pilots in the UK imply that another set of negotiations occurred within the teams which superseded the rational process of a scoring system. In these instances, the primary health care team decided to work on issues of lower priority either because they felt they already had a programme for action for the high-scoring items or because they felt overwhelmed and powerless to address the priority issue. This is a key lesson for PCGs to consider .

Primary care professionals need to be clear about the fundamental nature of health needs assessment. Needs assessment is a process concerned with making judgements of how to use scarce public money and the scarce professional resources available. So how should competing claims for health care resources be assessed and ranked? Equity is a central issue in resource allocation even within a small team. Equity can be concerned with financial and geographical equity, equity of service use, equity of treatment outcome, equity of health status, and equity of access to health services.[46] Horizontal equity aims to treat those with the same need equally, vertical equity is the aim of allocating more to those with greatest need.[47] Beliefs as to the 'fair' distribution of resources (and consequently the prioritization of issues to address) are influenced by differing viewpoints (egalitarian, entitlement, utilitarian) on distributive justice. These beliefs have a profound effect on the outcome of needs assessment. Beliefs which emphasize that resource distribution should maximize the benefit to the whole community – irrespective of who benefits– (utilitarian) can have a significant effect for older people, for example:

> 'that the strength of claims to health care resources should be assessed solely in terms of capacity to benefit has profound implications for older people ... For example units of measure such as 'quality adjusted life years' (QALYs) are as it were loaded against older people.'[48]

The government has named one of its priorities ' to improve the health of the worst off in society at a faster rate than the rest of the population'.[49] It has stated that targets should be identified in each health improvement programme for addressing local health inequalities. This has the potential for a more public exposure of the values that inform resource allocation decisions and consequently the value placed on health care for older people, for example:

> 'Lambeth, Southwark, and Lewisham Health Authority is prioritizing investment in the early years of life (by supporting mothers, babies, children, and young families) with the aim of producing the greatest long-term health benefit for the area's population. However, the Authority acknowledges that the aim of devoting more effort (and resources) to improving the health of younger people could be at odds with its other priorities, such as reducing disease and disability for older people'. [50]

HImPs have the potential for supporting the development of services for older people, although the value judgements made explicit in this statement may be replicated across the country. Each PCG has to contribute to determining a health authority-wide HImP[51] for the population. In the first year it has to address the following elements:

- two of the targets from the policy document *Our healthier nation*.[52] It should be noted that only one of the targets in this document addresses older people – perhaps an indication of the endemic lack of value placed on older people in health policies. Only the target of reducing the rate of accidents is directed at people over 75, all other targets specify people under 65.
- one target addressing local health inequalities. The guidance[53] gives examples of local objectives as fair access to services for black and ethnic minority groups, but again only mentions older people specifically in relation to the target for progress on reduction of accident rates
- targets from the joint improvement programme led by the local authority,[54] including:
  - reducing the rate of growth in emergency admissions to hospital of people aged 75 and over
  - developing a range of services to prevent or delay loss of independence for adults, including respite care

– ensuring systems are in place to identify carers and to provide them
with the support and services to maintain their health
– improving older people's opportunities for optimal recuperation and
rehabilitation through implementing specified proposals.[55]

Just as any health needs assessment at practice level will expose a discussion
about the values informing resource allocation, so will the development of
HImPs. Some methods of involving users in prioritizing health resources have
begun to be explored but require much more development and thought.[56]
Initiatives such as the citizens' jury or panels are providing one methodology
at a macro level.[57] However, there has been little exploration of how to specifically involve older people in these initiatives.

So far we have outlined the costs and challenges in undertaking a needs
assessment. But what are the benefits? Why should primary care teams consider undertaking this work specifically concerned with older people?

The evidence from developing countries shows that in situations of scarce
health resources drawing on the community itself in a COPC cycle provides
ways forward, but that changes are seen over 10–15 year periods.[58,59] The
COPC experience in the USA demonstrates changes in the way state-aided
primary care services are provided, and proponents point to its strength in
counterbalancing the excesses of the market–driven acute sector.[60] Some argue
that the evidence to support the application of the COPC model to primary
care in the UK is weak, and that primary care teams and PCGs need to consider methods that minimize the costs but maximize the benefits. So what are
the benefits of engaging in COPC-type processes in the UK? We argue that
these include:

• the ability to understand the wider picture of the influences and issues in
the health of older people in that practice or PCG
• the ability to keep some of the more strategic development issues in sight
rather than always focusing on short-term, crisis-driven solutions
• the ability to draw on a wider framework of solutions, including the community itself
• the ability to make underlying values concerning the health care of older
people explicit
• and, as a by-product, the value-added benefit of individuals networking
across agencies.

Questions for the primary care for older people research agenda

• What are the optimum ways of capitalizing on the information and
knowledge base from practices and local teams in health needs assessment
of older people without creating administrative data-collection night-
mares or futile isolated activities?
• How can primary care professionals support the process of meaningful
involvement of older people into health needs assessment processes?

Readers are invited to test these ideas out, in a paper exercise, by considering how they would tackle the health problems of any of the ageing ethnic minority populations in Britain. Until recently it has been assumed in the NHS that the size of the ethnic minority population aged, say, 75 years or more, was small and that local modification of services to meet the needs of the small number of individuals involved would occur. We should doubt whether the latter necessarily happens, but must also appreciate that the diverse ethnic minorities in Britain are ageing too, and if they have specific needs for, or perceptions of, care in later life, these will matter on a growing scale. The research literature on the health needs of ethnic minorities is scanty, at least in Britain, but we can start with some observations:

- The relatively good health of migrants wears off with time as ethnicity so often overlaps with social deprivation as a cause for illness and disability, but the patterns of morbidity in first-generation migrants tend to replicate those of the home country rather than the host.[61]
- Apparently straightforward issues may have profoundly different meanings – urinary frequency may suggest infection, diabetes, or detrusor instability to the white reader but may raise issues of privacy, hygiene, and religious observance when discussed with some Hindus, Sikhs, or Muslims.[62]
- Low uptake of community health and social services by ethnic minority elders may be interpreted differently by practitioners from different ethnic groups. White GPs may see low uptake as evidence for care by the extended family, whilst Asian GPs may see it as evidence of language barriers, limited knowledge of services, and poor service response.[63]
- Assumptions about family care made by gatekeepers may explain the under-representation of older black people on community nurse caseloads in the Midlands[64] and the underutilization of services for leg ulcers by ethnic minority elders in West London.[65.]
- Cultural diversity and disadvantage combine together in different ways for different ethnic minorities, suggesting that practitioners should avoid seeing ethnic minority elders as a 'problem group' and instead look for specific solutions to specific problems in particular populations.[66]

Given this background, how could the COPC approach be used to develop or reconfigure services for specific ageing ethnic minorities?

To summarize, we have argued that the provision of health and social care to older people is complex, competes for limited resources, and in many instances fails to provide the level of quality individual professionals would aspire to. If the services in primary care are to improve across the range it provides – from health promotion to care of the people who are dying at home – then there needs to be a systematic method of each team agreeing which are the most important areas to work on and improve. Health needs assessment in primary care has experimented with a multiplicity of approaches. The focus on PCGs and their constituent primary care teams allows for the first time the potential for symbiosis between the creativity of small teams and the responsibility for addressing issues of equity across wider populations. We move on to look at some of these issues of creativity and innovation in the next chapter.

References

1 NHSE Health Service Circular 1998/167 *Health improvement programmes: planning for better health and better health care.* Department of Health, London 1998.

2 Department of Health *Modernising health and social services: national priorities guidance 1990/00–2001/02.* DOH, London 1998.

3 Lawrence M & Packwood T Adapting total quality management for general practice: evaluation of a programme. *Quality in Health Care* 1996; **5**:151–8.

4 Gillam S & Miller R *Community-orientated primary care – a public health experiment in primary care.* King's Fund, London 1997.

5 Moss F Risk management and quality of care. *Quality in Health Care* 1995; **4**(2) 102–7.

6 Gillam S & Murray S *Needs assessment in general practice.* Occasional paper 73. Royal College of General Practice, London 1996.

7 See, for example, Williamson I & Pickin C The life-cycle framework, and Gabbay M & Gabbay J Assessing the needs of hard-to-reach groups in Harris A (ed.) *Needs to know: a guide to needs assessment in primary care.* Churchill Livingstone, London 1997.

8 Bradshaw J The concept of social need. *New Society* 1972; **30**:640–3.

9 Blaxter M *Consumer issues within the NHS.* NHS Executive Research and Development Directorate, 1995.

10 Jordan J & Wright J Making sense of health needs assessment. *British Journal of General Practice* 1997; **November**:695–6.

11 NHS Management Executive *Assessing health care needs.* DHA project discussion paper, EL(91) 41,1991.

12 Stevens A & Sadler A *Epidemiological-based needs assessment.* In Harris A (1997), op. cit.

13 Gillam S & Murray S *Needs assessment in general practice.* Occasional paper 73. Royal College of General Practice, London 1996.

14 Orr J Health visiting and the community. In Luker K & Orr J (eds) *Health visiting* Blackwell Scientific Publications, Oxford 1985.

15 Henderson P & Thomas D *Skills in neighbourhood work* . National Institute Social Services Library No. 39. George Allen & Unwin, London 1980.

16 Ashton J & Seymour H *The new public health.* Open University Press, Milton Keynes 1988.

17 Peckham S & Spanton J Community development approaches to health needs assessments. *Health Visitor* 1994; **67**(4):124–5.

18 Neve H Community assessment. Iin Burton B & Harrison L (eds) *Identifying local health needs* . Policy Press, University of Bristol 1996.

19 Murray S & Gillam S Community assessment for general practice. In Harris A (1997), op.cit.

20 Cernik K & Wearne M Using community health profiles to improve service provision. *Health Visitor* 1992; **65**:343–5.

21 Jones H & Dowrick C Assessing community care needs within general practice. *Health and Social Care in the Community* 1996; **4**(4):234–5.

22 Levenson R, Joule N, & Russell J Case study 15: the New River total care project. In *Developing public health in the NHS : the multidisciplinary contribution*. King's Fund, London 1997.

23 Cited in Neve H (1996), op. cit.

24 Murray S & Graham LJC Practice-based health needs assessment: use of four methods in a small neighbourhood. *British Medical Journal* 1995; **310**:1443–8.

25 Mackenzie I, Nelder R, & Radford G Needs assessment at a practice level: using routine data in a meaningful way. *Journal of Public Health Medicine* 1997; **19**(3):255–61.

26 Levenson R, Joule N, & Russell J Case study 16 : practice profiling in North Downs Community Trust. In *Developing public health in the NHS: the multidisciplinary contribution*. King's Fund, London 1997.

27 Patel D Primary care: the use of general practice computer systems. *In The benefits of using clinical information* pp.147–151. Enabling People Programme, IM & T Strategy, NHSE 1997.

28 Mitchell P Paris nexus: a community care and social services integrated information system. *Health Service Journal* 1998; **December**:4–5.

29 Allen I, Hogg D, & Peace S *Elderly people: choice, participation and satisfaction*. Policy Studies Institute, London 1992.

30 Illesly V, Goldstone L, & Ruxton L *District nursing monitor II* Unique Business Services Ltd, University of Northumbria, Newcastle 1993.

31 Department of Health *Involving patients examples of good practice* NHS Executive, Leeds 1996.

32 Murray S A, Tapson J, Tunrbull L, *et al.* Listening to local voices: adapting rapid appraisal to assess health and social needs in a general practice. *British Medical Journal* 1994; **308**:698–700.

33 Black D & Craig P Assessing health outside the health service. In Harris A (1997), Op. cit.

34 College of Health '*Ask the patient*'. Report on new approaches to consumer audit feedback in general practices. College of Health, London 1991.

35 See, for example, the listing given from 1980 onwards in Jones J *Community development and health education*. Roots and Branches Papers from the Open University /Health Education Authority Winter School on Community Development and Health, Open University, Buckingham. 1990.

36 Thornton P & Tozer R *Involving older people in planning and evaluating community care: a review of initiatives.* Social Policy Research Unit, University of York 1994.

37 Neve H Community assessment. In Burton B & Harrison L (eds) *Identifying local health needs.* Policy Press, University of Bristol 1996.

38 Pollock A & Majeed F Community-orientated primary care: not a panacea for the problems faced by primary care. *British Medical Journal* 1995; **310**:481–2.

39 Scobie S, Basnett I, & McCartny P Can general practice data be used for needs assessment and health care planning in an inner London district? *Journal of Public Health Medicine.* 1995; **17**(4):475–83.

40 OPCS *Morbidity statistics from general practice 1991–92.* Fourth National Study. HMSO, London 1995.

41 Health Education Authority *1992 Health and lifestyles surveys.* HEA, London 1994.

42 Health Education Authority *Health and lifestyles: black and minority ethnic groups in England.* Health Education Authority, London 1994.

43 Department of Health *The new NHS: primary care groups delivering the agenda.* Health Service Circular 1998/228.

44 Department of Health *Launch of review group to establish the new national framework on services for older people.* Press release. DoH, November 1998.

45 Gillam S & Miller R *Community-orientated primary care – a public health experiment in primary care.* King's Fund, London 1997.

46 Harris A & Marshall T The language of needs assessment. In Harris A (1997), op. cit.

47 Whitehead M *The concepts and principles of equity in health.* WHO Regional Office for Europe, Copenhagen 1990.

48 Howse K Health care rationing: non-treatment and euthanasia. In Bernard M & Philips J (eds) *The social policy of old age.* Centre for Policy on Ageing, London 1998.

49 Department of Health *Modernising health and social services: national priorities guidance 1990/00–2001/02.* Local Authority Circular (98) 22, NHSE 1998/159.

50 King's Fund *Local inequalities targets: discussion paper.* King's Fund, London 1998.

51 NHSE Health Service Circular 1998/167 op cit.

52 Department of Health *Our healthier nation.* Cm.3852. Stationery Office, London 1998.

53 Department of Health *Modernising Health and Social Services : national priorities guidance 1999/00–2001/02.* Local Authority Circular (98) 22, NHSE 1998/159.

54 Department of Health *Modernising health and social services : national priorities guidance 1999/00–2001/02*, pp.24–5. Local Authority Circular (98) 22, NHSE 1998/159.

55 Department of Health *Better services for vulnerable people – maintaining the momentum.* HSC 1998/139. Local Authority Circular (98) 21, annexe B, action 1. 1998.

56 Hopkins A, Gabbay J, & Neuberger J Role of users of health care in achieving quality service. *Quality in Health Care* 1994; **3**:203–9.

57 McIver S *Independent evaluation of citizens' juries in health authorities settings: executive summary.* King's Fund, London 1998.

58 Kark SL *Community-orientated primary health care.* Appleton-Century-Crofts, New York 1981.

59 Gillam S & Miller R Community-orientated primary care – a public health experiment in primary care. King's Fund, London 1997.

60 Wright P Community-orientated primary care: the cornerstone of health care reform. *Journal of the American Medical Association* 1993; **269**:2544–7. 1993

61 McKeigue P Patterns of health and disease in the elderly from ethnic minority groups. In Squires AJ (ed) *Multicultural health care and rehabilitation of older people.* Edward Arnold, London 1991.

62 Qureshi B Ethnic elders and the general practitioner. In Squires AJ (ed) *Multicultural health care and rehabilitation of older people.* Edward Arnold, London 1991.

63 ³Pharoah C *Primary health care for elderly people from black and ethnic minority communities.* Age Concern Institute of Gerontology, HMSO, London 1995.

64 Cameron E, Badger F, & Evers H District nursing, the disabled and the elderly: who are the black patients? *Journal of Advanced Nursing Studies* 1989; **14**:376–82.

65 Franks PJ, Morton N, Campbell A, *et al.* Leg ulceration and ethnicity: a study in West London. *Public Health* 1997; **111**:327–9.

66 Atkin K Ageing in multi-racial Britain: demography, policy and practice. In Bernard M & Phillips J (eds) *The social policy of old age* Centre for Policy on Ageing, London 1998.

CHAPTER TWELVE

Changing primary care for
older people

The previous chapter examined the process of health needs assessment for a population of older people. This chapter explores the issues in changing services and ends with an agenda for change for primary care groups.

Looking outward to a spectrum of innovation

A health needs assessment process identifies the problems in individuals and whole populations but a separate process is required to identify the most appropriate solutions. The pressures of the daily workload invariably make practitioners draw on their immediate knowledge in identifying solutions, rather than focus outward to use other sources for generating ideas and solutions. Without a wider perspective we are destined to fail to learn from past experience and ignore sources of potential creativity. The ethos of looking outward for knowledge is inherent in many current policy documents, for example in continuing professional education for doctors and nurses,[1] and is cited as an aspect of clinical governance.[2] The PCGs are charged with providing mechanisms which support this outward-looking approach through sharing innovations[3] and working in partnership with local authorities and the voluntary sector. NHS and local government beacon services are intended to share good practice with others through open days, secondments, and seminars, and by providing details for the database of Service Delivery Practice (SDP) currently being established on the NHS Intranet.[4] The introduction of a National Framework for service provision for older people[5] holds out the idea of a blueprint drawn from collective experience.

At a primary care team level, an outward-looking approach includes:

*   networking locally, professionally, and more widely
*   awareness of current developments and innovations in the field through reading relevant professional journals and attending continuing professional development educational events
*   actively searching for information through literature searches, approaches to professional organizations, and talking to people involved in the innovation elsewhere

- drawing on the experiences and ideas from other countries (as we discussed in Chapter 3).

This sort of approach takes both commitment and resources, with a risk of endless duplication of effort in, for example, undertaking literature searches. One means of capitalizing on resources and energy is to create links between the planning activities of the practice, the PCG, the community health services, and the local authority. Another is to create a database of local development activities as well as linked sources of evaluations of similar developments elsewhere. There have certainly been examples of databases of innovation in primary care at different times.[6] There are also examples of anthologies of innovation in the care of older people, often focused on a particular aspect such as health promotion.[7,8,9]

The challenge in primary care is to move from exciting ideas to sustainable implementation of service innovation. The experience over the first 50 years of the NHS is that innovation in primary care for older people has a number of features which the next 50 should seek to address:

- innovation has been widespread yet sporadic across the UK (see Chapter 1)
- evaluation of many of the innovations has been limited and consequently isolated in its impact, with little dissemination of the lessons
- much innovation has been dependent on fixed-term project funding and not absorbed into the mainstream when the project funding ends
- innovation driven from central government has resulted in widespread differences in implementation which cannot be explained in terms of differential health care needs of the local elderly population
- a narrow scientific paradigm imposed from the top downwards results in stagnation in service development (see Chapter 2).

It could perhaps be summed up by saying that for older people now there is little that is 'national' about the National Health Service, a situation that is all the more shocking when the critiques of services for older people in successive decades point to the same issues, irrespective of geographical location. To reiterate, these issues result from:

- the interplay of health and social problems for older people
- the territories, boundaries, divisions, and communication chasms between organizations and the professionals therein
- the failure to use a spectrum of professional skills and knowledge required to support the range of services in primary care provision – health promotion, acute care, continuing care, and care of people dying
- the reduction in use and availability of high-cost acute general hospital beds
- the failure to place enough priority on the health and care of older adults in the face of competition for resources and attention.

In the following section we provide an overview of organizational innovations that have been used to address these issues. This explores the range that a practice and PCG could consider in developing services. Pertinently, readers of this section are likely to have one or more of the following responses:

- 'that's an interesting idea'
- 'we're introducing that'
- 'that's not new – we've done or had that for the last five/ten/fifteen/twenty years'
- 'we *used* to provide that but the funding was withdrawn'
- 'we tried that, it didn't work so we stopped it'.

These serve to underline our comments about the nature of innovation and developments in health care for older people.

We have organized our overview into the issue categories given earlier in this chapter. We provide brief information but would not claim to be comprehensive in our listing as many of these types of innovations are never written up or publicized beyond the immediate locality.

Developments in addressing the interplay of health and social problems in promoting health and well-being

In this category we have identified five different types of initiatives:

1. The provision of *group sessions for health promotion and mutual support* in the health centre/practice setting.[10] Examples here include carers' groups as well as topic-based sessions such as smoking cessation. Many areas have had long traditions of more broad-based groups, such as pensioners health groups, which may have been run in primary care or within the local voluntary sector.[11]

2. *Alliances on exercise opportunities* for older people between primary care staff and Local Authority sports development staff have led to schemes such as prescription for exercise and exercise groups in primary care premises.[12]

Brief case example: t'ai chi and prescription for exercise for people over 60. A pilot scheme has been undertaken in Oldham, funded by the West Pennine Health Authority. t'ai chi, for which there is some evidence that it improves balance to prevent falls in older adults, is offered as one option in the prescription for exercise scheme on referral by practice nurses. Older people and key agencies were involved in the planning of this project. Age Concern provides the classes.[13]

3. The provision of *access to welfare benefits assessments and advice* through health centres and general practice.[14]

Brief case example. An advice worker was employed to provide a pro active outreach service on benefits/resource advice to practice patients aged over 80 in a general practice in London. Three hundred patients were offered financial need and benefits entitlement, particularly related to ill health and frailty. Only 5% were existing social service or Citizen's Advice Bureau clients. Of those who accepted the offer, the advice worker was able to increase annual benefit by £138 820 and gain one-off payments under the Social Fund or from charities to the total of £11 444 for immediate need such as fuel bills, funeral expenses, and purchasing furniture.[15] In addition, she was able to act as an advocate in getting landlords to deal with housing disrepair and safety issues in a number of cases.

4. The creation of multiple provision of facilities and services beyond sector boundaries and focused on local health needs – sometimes but not necessarily in one building. *Healthy Living Centres* are one such model which although not directed specifically at older adults, incorporate a range of health, local author-ity, and voluntary sector services.[16]

Brief case example: The West End Health Resource Centre in Newcastle-upon-Tyne was funded by the regional health authority, City Challenge, and Newcastle University. It took eight years to develop. A charitable trust holds management responsibility with membership from the local community as well as the council and health professionals. It houses a GP practice, chiropody, physiotherapy, speech therapy, health promotion, an integrated elderly care team, a 'rights pro-ject', a drug and alcohol support group, community room, crèche, gym, and com-plementary and family therapists.[17]

5. The provision of *community development workers in primary care settings* to assist or build community networks and activities related to health issues.[18]

Brief case example: The Wells Park Health Project has two community workers and is funded from the then FHSA. The project started in 1984, working closely with the Wells Park Practice. The project is a charity with a committee of local people including a GP and nurse from the practice. The activities are based on health needs assessment work from a lay perspective and consequent activities include welfare rights, housing advise and advocacy services, counselling services, group work with elders form ethnic minorities, exercise groups, reminiscence groups as well as a health library and equipment loan service.[19]

Using a spectrum of skill and knowledge bases to provide the range of services across primary care

In this section we identify seven different types of initiatives:

1. The *use of link workers and advocates*, most closely associated with elders whose first language is not English but used in other circumstances such as in older people with mental health problems. In a recent study of primary health care for elderly people from black and minority ethnic communities, the authors were able to report on the increased employment of link workers by FHSAs and general practices[20] available to assist in the provision of interpreting and advocacy.

2. The *use of volunteers* in a range of roles from good neighbour schemes to initial health assessment.[21] This includes the use of peers as health mentors and counsellors.[22]

> **Brief case example:** Devon Fair Exchange Project, an Ageing Well pilot project between Exeter and North Devon Health Authority and Age Concern Devon. A senior health mentors scheme was developed to address issues of isolation and consequent deterioration in mental health.[23] It aims to help older people by using peer group volunteers to encourage social activity and other aspects of health living. The national evaluation of this and other pilots is soon to be published.

3. The '*one-stop-shop*', *multiple health assessment and advice* in a clinic setting (with transport provided as necessary), with several different health professionals such as doctors, nurses, chiropodists, physiotherapists, audiologists, and dentists available for consultation. Examples of these include specifically for the housebound or as a method of targeting people over 75years old.[24]

> **Brief case example:** A series of one-stop health care workshops were offered to patients over 65 at the Manor Street Surgery, Hertfordshire. In this workshop the patient could consult the audiologist, chiropodist, occupational therapist, and social worker. The patients completed a self-report health questionnaire, received a health check by either the practice nurse, health visitor, or district nurse, together with flu immunization. Transport was provided through a community organization. The Women's Royal Voluntary Service (WRVS) with teenagers from the local school provided the reception service and refreshments.[25]

4. The provision of *consultant, specialist nurse, and professions allied to medicine (e.g. physiotherapist, dieticians, speech therapists, etc.) clinics in primary care* has expanded, particularly in the disease management of specific conditions such as diabetes. There are examples of consultant geriatricians providing similar outreach into primary care.[26] At the same time the expertise of primary care professionals has developed, increasing the amount of shared care between hospital teams and the primary care team. Other models have also developed in the provision of specialist clinics in primary care, such as the management of continence and leg ulcers,[27] using area-wide nurse specialists to support as well as train primary care professionals.

5. *The increased use of practice nurses and nurse practitioners to take a more prominent role in chronic disease management* – primarily the monitoring aspects. The introduction of legislation for nurse prescribing is relevant here but the omission of practice nurses without district nursing or health visiting qualifications from the scheme is likely to reduce its impact on chronic disease management for older people. The potential to take on an increased proactive case-finding and case management function by nurses is being explored in many ways. These include in pilots under the Primary Care Act 1998,[28] through the expansion of nurse practitioners roles[29] and through specific research trials.[30]

6. The *employment of health professionals (particularly community nurses) as*

community care managers by local authorities to use their knowledge base in commissioning and managing care packages for people.[31] Exploration of a wide range methods to engage health professionals in the process has been a feature of the nineties. A pilot in Derbyshire explored the role community pharmacists could take.[32]

> **Brief case example** In the implementation phase of the Community Care Act, funding was used to pilot the role of a district nurse care manager in the London Borough of Islington. This pilot identified that the district nurse was able to co-ordinate detailed assessment, care planning, and purchase of care for those people who had the most complex physical, medical, and social care needs very effectively. In addition she was viewed as a valuable resource for both her clinical knowledge and her understanding of the local health care systems to the social services care manager team.[33] Subsequently the London Borough of Islington funded five district nurse care managers (from the community health services) to work in their service.

7. The provision of a *designated health visitor or nurse for promoting and co-ordinating health care for older people in a practice population.*[34] More than any other developments listed, this will be the one to evoke the highest level of reader response as outlined above. Arguments for and against these types of posts have been made based on several interlocking issues, dependent often on the local resource climate. The first is the debate whether primary care nurses should be specialists or generalists. This argument could equally be applied to GPs and have been cyclical in social workers since the inception of social service departments. The second has hinged on the potential nebulous nature of the function – offering scope for differently trained people to provide part of it. The variety in the provision of the over 75 assessment (see Chapter 1) together with the designation of social workers as the care managers for older people has also affected these debates.

Addressing the boundary divisions and communication problems at the interface between organizations and professionals

In this section we identify six groupings of innovations:

1. Creating *liaison posts* to smooth or manage the transition for older people between one service and another. Most typically these have existed as posts from the community nursing service working within a hospital setting.[35] Other examples are of hospital-based discharge coordinators. In primary care, nurse liaison posts have been created by GP fundholders to promote smooth transition for their patients between a number of services, including into nursing homes.[36]

2. *The co-location of professionals and services* demonstrated through the provision of 'one-stop shops' for people in assessment clinics and shared premises (described above). Other examples are the co-location of the professionals' office bases, as Chapter 3.

3. The provision of *a single workforce of care assistants* who provide all

nursing, personal care, and domestic services to an older person with complex support needs in their own home.[37] Many of these innovations were in the period leading up to the implementation of the Community Care Act and then disappeared as budgetary demarcation became firmly defined.

4. The *provision of multi-agency and multiprofessional education* on aspects of health and social care of older people. Many of these examples are linked to specific issues discussed in Chapter 3.

5. *The development of explicit, local written descriptions of care processes involving different agencies and sectors*, such as care pathways, shared-care protocols, and joint operational policies.[38] The purpose of such written agreements are to improve coordination, collaboration, and effectiveness. The imperative of this type of clarity across the health and social care boundary comes not just from the experiences of delay in provision of care while the arguments rage over whether, for example, 'it's a health bath or a social care bath', but the reality for the older person in that personal care provided by the local authority is subject to means testing while care provided through health authority funding is free at the point of receipt. The Royal Commission on Long-term Care has recommended that all intimate personal care be provided free, subject to assessment of need but irrespective of provider. We look forward to implementation of this approach by the government.

Brief case example: *The wavy line: home care and community nursing working together* is a joint publication between Birmingham City Council Social Services Department and Birmingham Health Authorities and Trusts. It incorporates a set of agreements/protocols as to how the two services should work together in providing personal care to people in their own homes. It also provides criteria to make judgements as to when it is the responsibility of one service or the other.[39]

Addressing the reduction in the use/availability of high-cost hospital beds in the acute sector and in continuing care

In this we identify three types of innovation:

1. The provision of a *24-hour district nursing service*. The Audit Commission report on district nursing[40] demonstrates how variable the provision of nursing services are – in some parts of the country not available after five o' clock in the evening. This inequity of access to service provision demonstrates the question mark in the *national* nature of the NHS.

2. The development of *short-term, high-level rehabilitation, nursing, and social care support packages* for older people to allow them to leave hospital earlier post-surgery or acute episodes or to prevent their admission. These are forms of Hospital at Home schemes. The central government-funded 'Winter Crisis' moneys of 1997/1998/1999 gave a massive impetus to the development of rapid response teams and other schemes.[41,42]

Brief case example: North West Anglia Health Authority funded a rapid response nursing team in 1997. The aim was to prevent hospitalization of people by providing emergency services in the community for up to 72 hours. In the first six months the team cared for 101 people at home and 54 in designated nursing-home beds. The mean age of the patients was 79 and the main reasons for referrals were chest infections, pneumonia, and the need for support following an injury.[43]

3. The development of *intermediate care services through small in-patient units with GP medical cover.* The debates over the viability of GP-led community hospitals in rural areas has been present for the last 30 years.[44] There are examples of them in urban areas[45,46] These innovations have seen further exploration[47] with central government funding to avoid the cyclical winter bed crisis. There are also possibilities of funding this type of care, as well as respite care, in the burgeoning private nursing home sector.

Brief case example: An intermediate nurse-led care unit has been established at the Sir Alfred Jones Memorial Hospital, Liverpool. It provides in-patient care services for patients of GPs who need clinical respite, palliative care, or rehabilitation. It also provides care for patients who no longer need acute hospital facilities but are not ready to be discharged home.[48] In Solihull, the Grove Road General Practice, a total purchasing project, agreed with the local authority to jointly fund a bed in a nursing home for patients who needed nursing but not hospital care on a short-term basis. The health funding covered the first two weeks , by which time alternative provision would have been established or social services funding for the long term found.

Options for development

So against what criteria will a primary care team or a PCG consider these options for developments? In some instances the normal service provided over many years in one area would be considered an innovation in another, e.g. evening and night district nursing services. The absence of easily available descriptive data on structure, process, outcome and costs of such 'normal services' – data that during the period of the NHS 'internal market' became closely guarded business information not to be shared with potential competitors – is a not insignificant obstacle for PCGs. The lack of meaningful comparative data sets and commissioning (previously known as contract) currencies will continue to hamper PCGs as they try to consider which innovations to prioritize. In addition, the lack of common evaluative techniques for small-scale innovations makes it difficult to create a cumulative body of evidence. Innovation in service is an experiment, but not one where all the variables can be controlled to examine the effect of one. Consequently the evaluative activities often have multiple elements in order to consider context, structure, process, and outcome. In many instances it is comparative strategies in evaluation which add weight to the findings – comparison in terms of before and after the intervention, or comparison with similar innovations, or comparison with older people's experiences who have not been involved in the innovation. It would seem, however that the more the evaluation relies on the work of the service innovator, the more unlikely there is to be a comparative element, a point which PCGs should note in considering evaluative research of innovation.

Understanding change

Developing and improving services is about change. Change is exciting and dynamic for some people, energy sapping for others, and plain terrifying for a few. Many primary care professionals have experienced multiple, rapid work-related changes in the past 10–15 years. Often they describe themselves as 'change weary', desperate for stability while recognizing that is unlikely in societies grappling with economic imperatives, technological advances, and demographic shifts. So what do we understand about making changes and how can we use that in our agendas for health and social care for older people?

Any change process has five parts:[49]

(1) precipitating factors
(2) the members' felt need for change
(3) decisions/plans for instigating change
(4) implementation
(5) outcomes (intended and unintended).

The precipitating factors come from within or without a team. This could be anything from the experience of one patient (such as death at home undiscovered for a considerable time) or the publication of a systematic review of evidence for treatments such as the use of laxatives by older people.[50] Recent experience, however, demonstrates that legislation linked to finance has been a powerful precipitating factor for much of the change in primary care. These precipitating factors have then to be accepted by the members and expressed as a need to change. The tension here is that all members do not necessarily accept the precipitating factors. However, once a sufficiently powerful group of individuals within a organization feel the need to change, plans are then made which inevitably involve change for part or all of the organization. Almost all changes in organizations face resistance from individuals and groups. The four most common reasons people resist change are

(1) a desire not to lose something of value
(2) a misunderstanding of the change and its implications
(3) belief that the change does not make sense for the organization
(4) low tolerance for change.[51]

Decision-making and planning change therefore has to include a number of elements. The participation of people in different positions in the organization is important as well as leadership with energy, commitment, and authority (either because of their position, e.g. a partner in the practice, or conferred by an authoritative body like the practice executive). The planning has to capitalize on the energy and ideas of those supporting the change as well as reduce the resistance to the change. Lewin's Force Field[52] is a commonly cited model (Figure 12.1) used in analysing a situation in order to try to get as much energy as possible behind the change and as little energy as possible resisting it. He argued that the best strategy for implementing change was to reduce the restraining forces as unilateral increases in driving forces only met with an equal and opposite increase in resistance to change.

Another way of thinking of this is to consider what each person or group might be saying if you stood in their shoes and viewed the proposed change. Resistance to change can be at the individual, the group, or organizational level. Strategies for reducing restraining forces resistance include:[53]

- inviting resisters to participate in the planning and implementation
- widening the dissemination of proposals and consultation processes in the organization
- demonstrating commitment to modify the proposals within the parameters of the objectives as a result of the consultation
- developing alternative plans
- wearing out the resistance over time.

In summary, the energy for change has to be maximized so that it is greater than the perceived cost of changing. The energy comes from the felt need for change, together with a clarity of the intended change and the practical steps to reach it. While detailed planning of the pragmatic steps for change is clearly essential, so too is an implementation process which allows the participants to feedback and modify the plans in the light of experience and other events.

The following primary care team-level case study illustrates some of these elements.

Following an investigation of incidence and management of continence in the practice population (undertaken by a practice nurse as part of her studies for a post-registration qualification), one GP (of five partners) and the practice nurse agree they wish to address the issue of improving incontinence management in the practice for people over 65. Their first steps were to investigate how this was

Figure 12.1 Lewin's Force Field.

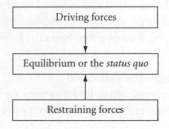

247

being done elsewhere by talking to a specialist continence nurse, requesting a literature search at their professional organizations' libraries, and through their local MAAG. They present both the practice nurse's study and some of their findings from their explorations at a lunch-time practice meeting of the whole team. They subsequently draw up a proposal for the partners' meeting which includes:

(1) the introduction of improved questions to identify continence problems in the over-75 assessment procedures
(2) the introduction of a computerized prompt for continence-problem questions annually for everyone over 65
(3) the development of a protocol and pathway detailing investigations and management linked to named people and services
(4) the introduction of a more significant role for the practice nurse team in conducting continence assessments, giving education and advice, as well as ordering continence management products such as pads and pants and following up patients with continence problems six-monthly
(5) producing publicity on the availability of the practice nurses for consultation on continence problems and briefing the reception staff and extended primary care team on this service change.

The proposal leads to a heated debate between the partners on issues of priorities and overload. The senior partner is unconvinced of the scale of the problem and refuses to entertain the idea of computerized prompts. Another partner is concerned about the workload implications for the practice nurses, detracting from their other duties which relate directly to income for the practice.

The GP and the nurse go away and work on a modified proposal. They also discuss the issue and ideas with the district nurses and health visitors. They discover one of the district nurses has completed specialist training in continence management and is keen to put her knowledge to greater use. A revised proposal is developed – it still includes items 1 and 3 but item 2 has been dropped. It now proposes a pilot of three months to investigate the feasibility of item 4. For this period only one practice nurse would be involved. In addition the district nurse would provide one hour a week for specific continence appointments in the surgery. The pilot would allow time to collect information on workload, outcomes, and consequences. The patients could either self-refer or be referred by a member of the team. Item 5 was adapted to reflect the change in the proposed item 4. The partners' meeting agreed the new pilot proposal.

The time chart in Figure 12.2 demonstrates the planning required in implementation and the length of time needed.

While resistance to change is a major issue and planning to reduce it is important, there are other internal and external factors that influence the success of implementing change. Analysis in the business world shows that the main barriers to achieving change come from the following or a combination of the following:[54]

• more time was needed than allocated
• major problems surfaced which had not been anticipated
• coordination of important activities was not effective

Figure 12.2 Case study implementation chart

Activity with name of individual	Month								
	1	2	3	4	5	6	7	8	9
1. Agree new questions for over-75s assessment with all who do the checks	✓								
2. Agree with practice administrator how and when they will be incorporated in documentation/computer	✓								
3. Draft and consult on protocol and supplementary information	✓	✓							
4. Agree with practice manager method of production of protocol		✓							
5. Launch of new protocol and new questions accompanied by a practice lunch and enthusiast guest speaker from specialist/secondary services			✓						
6. Identify times and venue for district nurse consultations with practice	✓								
7. Agree data collection items and methods for both the introduction of key questions and the three-month pilot		✓							
8. Any additional training and knowledge needs of nurses addressed		✓	✓						
9. Administrative team briefed on purpose and method of pilot			✓						
10. Patient publicity agreed and produced			✓						
11. Launch of pilot services				✓					
12. Feedback meetings between nurses and lead GP				✓	✓	✓	✓		
13. Evaluation report of pilot produced for partner's meeting and linked with community health service manager							✓		
14. Protocol reviewed in team clinical meeting								✓	
15. Evaluation report of additional questions in assessment									✓
16. Proposals made for future changes and wider dissemination of the experiences									✓

- competing activities and crises distracted attention
- the skills and abilities of employees involved in the change was not sufficient
- training and support to lower-level employees was inadequate
- powerful external events interfered.

Most readers will find some resonance with the list in their own experiences. Practices, community health services, and PCGs should note this list in drawing up the agenda for developing primary and community health services. The complexity of health and social services, combined with competing issues demanding attention, make it ripe ground for most changes to falter on at least one of these barriers.

The following case study reflection on the introduction of research-based evidence in the management of leg ulcers also provides lessons in change management for PCGs.

The leg ulcer tale

Leg ulcers are a common, chronic, unpleasant, recurring condition. Estimates are that 1.5–3 people per 1000 population have active leg ulcers with an increase to 20 people per 1000 aged above 80,[55] in a female/male ratio of approximately 7:1. Associated pain, odour, and immobility contributes to social isolation and depression.[56] The aetiology of chronic leg ulcers is multifactorial but strongly associated with venous disease while arterial disease is present in approximately 20% of cases (some in conjunction with venous disease). Healing rates are problematic – some people having active ulceration for years – 60 years is documented in one instance.[57] Not only are they difficult to heal but re-occurrence is commonplace with rates quoted as high as 69%[58] in those with previous deep vein thrombosis or unable to comply with compression stockings. Annual costs to the NHS were estimated as between £230–400 million in 1991, of which nursing time was a major element.[59]

Most people with leg ulcers are managed by GPs and community nurses, with a uneven pattern of use of secondary services. In primary care the management of leg ulcers is often seen as an area of nursing expertise – not least because about a fifth of any district nursing caseload will be made up of patients with leg ulceration, estimated to account for up to half of their patient contact time.[60] In the late eighties the work from the Riverside community leg ulcer clinics began to be published.[61] This demonstrated that the combined effect of the following could significantly improve healing rates to 70% within 12 weeks:

- a centralized, specialist community leg ulcer clinic staffed by well-trained nursing staff
- differentiation of arterial and venous leg ulcers through the use of Doppler ultrasound
- application of best evidence in wound management techniques
- high compression bandaging achieved through four layers, developed in Charing Cross Hospital, London.

The potential benefit to patients and district nursing services was self-evident and was spelt out in publications in the early 1990s.[62] There followed a period where district nursing services across the country tried a variety of models[63] to replicate these results. These included community nurse-run clinics, community hub and spoke models with vascular surgeons at the hub clinics, and education and training of all district nursing sisters and practice nurses in Doppler assessment and four-layer bandaging – a range of activity spurred not least by the only Department of Health endorsed[64] clinical guidance applicable to nursing.[65] In the health authority contracts for district nursing this became used as a quality specification, often with specified healing rates – one of the few tangible clinical-effectiveness targets in community nursing with clear criteria for audit as specified in the nationally recommended audit tool. [66] Many of these experiences were difficult for reasons which are valuable to reflect on. They included:

- issues of how to gain and retain both competence and confidence in the diagnostic and bandaging techniques arose for many district nurses and practice nurses
- the impracticality for some nurses, such as practice nurses undertaking systematic initial assessment processes which could take up to an hour
- debates of value of a small number of the expert nurses versus the generalist community nurse took place
- the investment and revenue costs in both portable Doppler equipment and initially some of the expensive bandages (now only the orthopaedic wool padding) – not available through FP10s and not obviously recouped through savings in a reduced nursing workload – created barriers to implementation in some areas
- emulating the venous ulcer healing rates of the initial research team was only possible with strict exclusion of non-venous ulceration and people unwilling to use high-compression bandages.

The development and implementation of evidence-based guidance has continued throughout the nineties. In 1997 a systematic review of compression therapy for venous leg ulcers was published,[67] followed in 1998 by clinical practice guidelines for nurses in the management of patients with venous leg ulcers as part of a national sentinel audit project funded by the Department of Health.[68] Research continues to investigate the many unanswered aspects, e.g. a recent randomized controlled trial has shown centralized provision in community clinics to have improved healing rates over normal practice by district nurses[69] and the national Health Technology Assessment Programme has commissioned an RCT into the efficacy and cost-effectiveness of different methods of high-compression bandaging. The recent national review of district nursing services produced very critical data of the non-application of evidence-based practice in the assessment and care of leg ulcers by district nurses across seven community trusts.[70] While not decrying the range of excellent work that has been done to improve the spread of evidence-based nursing practice in wound and leg ulcer management, the issues cited above illustrate some of the pitfalls of narrowly applying best evidence into the lives of older people and primary care professionals.

We would like to outline two further issues:

(1) While healing rates for venous leg ulcers have improved in many areas, the rate of re-occurence has not changed. Class 3 compression stockings

reduces re-occurrence rates when compared with class 2 stockings, but are poorly tolerated. [71] This suggests that other lateral thinking needs to be applied to developing other preventative or treatment options. It certainly indicates that the reduction in personal and service costs will not be of the order dreamed of in the early nineties. Certainly there are vascular surgeons arguing that initial assessment by specialists using duplex scanning could improve outcomes for patients – rather than referring to vascular surgeons when the person has recurring ulcers embedded in chronic scar tissue. [72] Is this a bid in a turf war or a question PCGs should consider seriously?

(2) Aspects of the most clinically effective practice are unacceptable to some older people. There are widely quoted anecdotal examples of older people not complying with their treatment regime because a healed ulcer may mean they lose the social contact. [73] Some people find the bandages and their pressure intolerable for whatever reason – so they loosen them, poking knitting needles in to scratch the surrounding skin, or take them off to let the air in. Nurses often find themselves negotiating and bargaining with the older person to achieve compromise between what the person sees as quality-of-life issues and what the nurse knows is the most effective practice. In the case of wound healing this will include everything from elevating their leg, which will increase pain for some people but will aid venous return, to using a more flexible form of bandaging which will decrease the healing rate but allow the person to have baths.

In developing a clinical governance agenda, implementing, training for, and auditing clinical guidance on the management of chronic leg ulcers seems a straightforward option, however we would caution PCGs to think about the issues illustrated above and consider the resources available to consider the condition in its totality as well as a whole systems response.

The PCG agenda for improving primary care services for older people

So given our debates so far, what would we propose during this period of genesis of primary care groups? To remind ourselves, PCGs are charged with three main functions:

(1) health improvement – through the Health Improvement Programme
(2) primary and community health service development – through clinical governance, management of prescribing budgets (including the introduction of nurse prescribing), and primary care investment plans
(4) to advise on or commission secondary care services – through service and financial frameworks.

Health improvement plans

Figure 12.3 provides an overview of their content and process. Primary care group priorities for action are identified from the National Priorities for

Figure 12.3 *The Health Improvement Programme 'Cycle'.*[76]

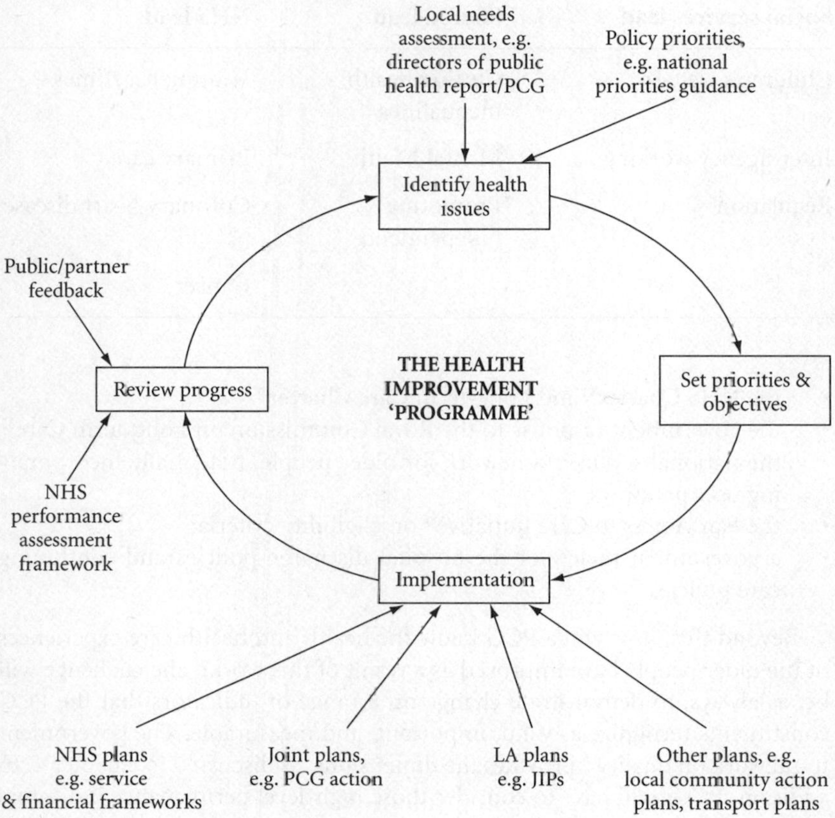

Health and Social Services,[74] other related national guidance, and their local needs assessment. These are worked into local objectives which address both the government White Paper *Saving lives: our healthier nation*[75] and joint action on the health and social care boundary determined through elements of the local authority-led joint investment plan. In the maze of central government policy guidance, we found it helpful to try and identify those objectives of specific relevance to older people.

The government determined national priorities for health and social services are shown in Table 12.1[77] below.

Since the publication of the national priorities, other White Papers and central government guidance have provided more specific detail on objectives which we incorporate in the listing below. A quick look at these objectives allows us to write a shopping list of issues that need to be thought about, using the information from earlier chapters. We produce this in a table format for ease of reading (Table 12.2).

Scanning the horizon there are a number of central initiatives which are likely to impact further on this shopping list. These include:

Table 12.1 *Government-determined national priorities for health and social services[77]*

Social services lead	Shared lead	NHS lead
Children's welfare	Cutting health inequalities	Waiting list /times
Inter-agency working	Mental health	Primary care
Regulation	Promoting independence	Coronary heart disease
		Cancer

- the NHS Charter[83] and Long-term Care Charter[84]
- the government response to the Royal Commission on Long-term Care[85]
- the national service framework for older people, potentially incorporating user pathways
- the Fair Access to Care initiative[86] on eligibility criteria
- a government review of the hospital discharge policies and continuing care policies.[87]

Beyond this, how will a PCG know the health and health care experiences of the older people have improved as a result of this work? The challenge will be, as always, to demonstrate change on a range of indicators that the PCG constituents recognize as valid, important, and measurable. The government framework on quality[88] provides the dimensions, as discussed in Chapter 4. In addition, PCGs will have to consider those high-level performance indicators which will be generated nationally, such as the rate of emergency admission for complications in asthma, epilepsy, and diabetes. The one given below relates specifically to older people:[89]

High level quality indicator	Explanation
Delayed discharge from hospital for people aged 75 or over , per 1,000 of those aged 75 or over and not in hospital	This interfaces with the Personal Social Services Performance Framework. Hospital discharge marks the boundary between numerous care organisations. Delayed discharge may be the result of poor communication between the relevant care organizations

How will PCGs decide what the important issues are, and where should they begin? It would seem that PCGs and local authorities are being inundated with policy guidance on a massive change agenda with timetables geared to the parliamentary electoral cycle. Reflecting on our brief descriptions on why

Table 12.2

National objectives	Possible actions
1. Cutting health inequalities objectives	
1.1 Develop action programmes to address areas of particular local health inequality, e.g. poverty and illness	A third of the retired population live on very low incomes, and their lives can be changed significantly through targeted benefits advice.
1.2 Reduce the rate of accidents by 20% by 2010 from a baseline at 1996	Prevention of falls in older people is a key issue. Multifactorial interventions are necessary, as outlined in Chapter 5, including physical exercise promotion, medication review, assessment of enviromental hazards, and consideration of alcohol consumption.
1.3 Reducing smoking prevelance	Respiratory disease contributes to the high prevelance of disability in older age groups. Smoking cessation is beneficial but often dismissed as a possibility with older people (see Chapter 10).
2. Mental health objectives	
Improve users and carers' access to services, the quality of continuing care and treatment they receive, and reduce the death rate from suicide by at least a fifth	The agenda is obvious (see Chapter 9): • a wider range of responses to depression in later life • earlier recognition of dementia • closer working with specialists in response to psychotic illness in old age.
3. Promoting independence objectives	
3.1 Prevent or delay loss of independence by developing and targeting a range of preventative services for adults, including respite care	Establish a minimal assessment and prevention programme for older people with clear, clinical case management responsibilities (Chapter 3) and clarity of access into the local authority services identified under their 'preventative strategy'[78] for this purpose.

Table 12.2 *Continued*

National objectives	Possible actions
3.2 Provide carers with the support and services to maintain their health and with the information they need on the health status and medication of the person they are caring for (subject to that person's consent). Ensure that systems are in place in primary care and in social services. Authorities to identify patients and service users who are, or who have, carers	Local authorities have the lead in implementing the National Carers' Strategy[79] which is set to stimulate more carer support services, including the provision of short breaks. A key element will be ensuring primary health care professionals are aware of the services and the mechanisms for directing carers to them.
3.3 Reduce nationally the per capita growth in emergency admissions of people aged over 75 to an annual average of 3% over five years	Local examination of information regarding reasons for emergency admission in order to determine issues to address, which could include increased availability of alternate care services (see earlier in this chapter for examples).
3.4 Improve older people's opportunities for optimal recuperation and rehabilitation by implementing the proposals in *Better services for vulnerable people*[80]	This includes the local review of the effectiveness of current arrangements for multidisciplinary assessments of people with complex needs against the recommendations of two national reports *The coming of age*[81] and *Investing in rehabilitation*[82]

4. Primary care objectives

National objectives	Possible actions
4.1 Reduce inequalities in access to NHS dentistry	Dental problems affect physical and emotional well-being, not least nutritional status and self-image. For those older people with low incomes and high levels of disability, the development of creative opportunities such as one-stop shop services, including dental, may need consideration.
4.2 Set targets to achieve more equal access for patients of high-quality standards of general practice in terms	Monitoring access of older patients to practices, reviewing need for home visiting, auditing care of

of clinical care, speed, convenience, and range of integrated services close to home

4.3 Set local targets to increase the level of generic prescribing and achieve, a reduction in the level of antibiotic prescribing

common conditions, and establishing case management for older people.

The issues for improving prescribing for older people are set out in Chapter 3, and include:
• addressing the undertreatment of certain conditions
• targeting regular medicine review on those in receipt of three or more medications, and on key drug groups that generate iatrogenesis.

5. Cardiovascular disease and stroke objectives

Begin to plan for the achievement of the proposed *Saving lives: our healthier nation* target – a reduction in the death rate from coronary heart disease and stroke among people under 75

the agenda for older people is clear (see Chapter 7):
• optimal treatment of AF
• use of ACE inhibitors in heart failure
• smoking cessation
• use of aspirin after MI and stroke.

6. Cancer objectives

Action to contribute to the achievement of the proposed *Saving lives* target – the reduction in death from cancer among people under 75

Most malignancies occur with increasing prevalence as ageing occurs, but does a focus on cancer care – earlier diagnosis, intervention, and palliative care – have a specific old-age dimension?

7. Sexual health objectives – part of the White Paper *Saving lives*

Will the sexual health of older people be an issue at all for PCGs? Even in the debates around the costs of treatment for impotence?

8. Alcohol objectives – part of the White Paper Saving lives

How to increase awareness of the role this may play in other health problems such as falls; and will issues such as access to specialist alcohol and substance misuse services for older people be taken on by PCGs?

innovations fail earlier in the chapter, many professionals and managers will yet again be trying to steer a course which precludes burn-out but makes the most of the opportunities.

We suggest that the solutions to these problems lie in the implementation of the health needs assessment process and clinical governance in PCGs and in the working units of community-based services, whether general practices or community nursing teams. The ways in which clinical governance evolves will determine whether it succeeds or fails.

Clinical governance is about improving the quality of services by creating an environment in which excellence will flourish whilst making individuals accountable for standard setting, and for maintaining and monitoring performance. The dangers of combining a drive for high standards with a system of accountability – ultimately connected to revalidation or re-accreditation of professional workers – are:

- Clinical governance will be made too complicated and will overwhelm all concerned. The complexity of health problems in later life, with the overlap of organic, psychological, and social problems, make primary care for older people a challenging task. Attempting to document everything, to use standardized instruments to measure function and mental state for all, and to audit all aspects of care will result in disillusionment and failure. Being selective in addressing problems will be important for the survival of practitioners.
- The measures proposed could become excessively bureaucratic with substantial opportunity costs but with little effect on the quality of care. The 75-and-over check is an example of this, and we should learn the negative lesson that it teaches.
- The imposition of clinical standards from above will inevitably be met with some resistance, especially when the evidence base for them is thin.
- Organizations will move too quickly (or will reinvent the wheel) and leave many people – patients especially – way behind, not understanding what is happening.
- The climate of 'blame & shame' could become a disaster for clinical governance, reducing the willingness of practitioners to experiment and innovate. General practitioners who worry about being sued by angry relatives after they encourage an older patient to exercise more, and she falls and fractures her hip, are not likely to remain protagonists for physical activity.
- Rigid protocols and standards will be adopted that will not be achievable because they fail to appreciate that concepts of health and illness are flexible and variable (see, for example, the leg ulcer tale), and that acceptance of disability will vary from one individual to another.
- clinical governance will become a gesture, like so much else in the NHS, with glossy brochures full of statistics demonstrating success being produced by organizations that do less and less for patients.

Clinical governance that will be relevant to an older population will grow out of existing activities, including:

- Audit that is comprehensive, systematic, effective, and good value for money, such as measuring the impact of influenza immunization efforts identifying the shortfall, and remedying it
- implementation of evidence-based practice of the kind outlined for cardiovascular disease as described in Chapter 7
- risk management so that practitioners feel that they can identify and learn from mistakes (such as Mrs K.'s story), and aim to reduce risks (as far as possible in an inherently risky business). Iatrogenic diseases (those made by medication or medical intervention) are a prime target (see Chapter 3)
- quality assurance as an integral part of team effectiveness, including monitoring mechanisms, approaches to poor performance, and public involvement (see Chapter 4).
- Staff and organizational development to foster an environment which enables and encourages best practice at all times. This applies not only to clinical and professional practice but to the fundamental attitudes to age and ageing that we discussed in Chapter 1.

How can this approach be brought together with the HImP shopping list and made into real change in the way services function for older people? What mechanisms do we have for re-engineering primary care, given the failure of previous efforts?

One possibility is to adopt health needs assessment processes which engage many stakeholders but involves practitioners locally in determining the *priorities* for change within the constraints of the national guidance. The circular, reflective model in the community-orientated primary care approach recently explored by the King's Fund, as shown in Figure 12.4, holds one possibility:

- a broadly-based agreement about what needs to change ('community diagnosis')
- discussion of priorities
- careful planning for local change
- systematic implementation and monitoring
- a return to review original ideas where necessary.

Within a PCG there is still much to explore about the most effective methods for engaging all constituents in priorities for change. Techniques such as consensus development conferences, nominal group processes, Delphi techniques, and rapid appraisal have much to offer in this area, not least in generating the energy and commitment to undertaking the changes at individual and group levels. This is the exact opposite of the 'command and control' approach, in which decisions are taken and must be carried out without the opportunity to revisit and review them.

Primary health care for older people in the 21st century has all the lessons from the 20th to learn from, the new technologies to address old problems, and the potential for truly creative change. We hope that this book will assist practitioners of all disciplines to learn the lessons, apply the approaches, and achieve change for the benefit of all of us who hope to grow old in the 21st century.

Figure 12.4 *A model of community-oriented primary care.*

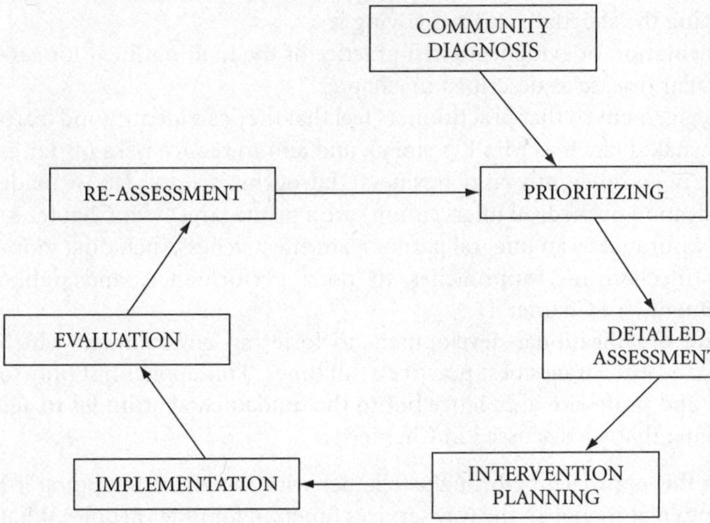

References

1 See, for example, the United Kingdom Central Council for Nursing, Midwifery and Health Visiting *The future of professional practice – the council standards for education and practice following registration* UKCC,1994.

2 Department of Health First Class Service *Quality in the new NHS*. Health Services circular 1998/113.

3 Health Services circular *The New NHS, modern and dependable: establishing a primary care group*. Department of Health 1998/065.

4 Cm 4320 Government Response to Health Committee *First report on the relationship between health and social services*: session 1989–1999. The Stationery Office, London 1999.

5 Department of Health press release on the reference group for setting standards of the NHS care for older people national service framework 1998/0597.

6 Harrison L & Neve H *A review of innovations in primary care*. The Policy Press, University of Bristol 1994.

7 Day L *Health visiting and older people*. Health Education Authority, London 1987.

8 Ageing Well. *Health Promotion with older people*. Age Concern, England. 1994.

9 Flanagan C & Barnes G *Health opportunities for older people in the North West*. A special report for the Regional Director of Public Health. University of Liverpool and North West Regional Task Force for Older People 1998.

10 Rebak A Setting up a 60 plus group in a health centre. *Community Health Action* 1994; **34**(13).

11 Tedesco D Exercise for the elderly in a rural community. *Health Visitor* 1997; **70**(1):32–3.

12 Fox K, Biddle S, Edmunds L, *et al*. Physical activity promotion through primary health care in England. *British Journal of General Practice*. 1997; **47**(419):367–9.

13 Flanagan C Accidents in older people. 1998 In Flanagan C & Barnes G (eds) *Health opportunities for older people in the North West* A special report for the Regional Director of Public Health. University of Liverpool and North West Regional Task Force for Older People, 1998.

14 Paris D & Player D Citizens advice in general practice. *British Medical Journal* 1993; **306**: 1518–20.

15 Mercer L. *Benefits advice to older people in a practice population*. Unpublished report, Innovative primary care for older people in Camden and Islington project, 1999.

16 Hogg C *Healthy living centres*. Department of Health, London 1998.

17 Davies J Super-models in practice. *Health Service Journal* 1998; **108**:6–8.

18 Jones J Community development and health education. *In Roots and Branches: papers from the Open University /Health Education Authority Winter School on Community Development and Health*. Open University, Buckingham 1990.

19 The Wells Park Health Project. Reported in Freeman R, *et al. Community development and involvement in primary care*. King's Fund, London 1997.

20 Pharoah C *Primary health care for elderly people from black and minority ethnic communities*. HMSO, London 1995.

21 Carpenter GI & Demopoulos GR Screening the elderly in the community: controlled trial of dependency surveillance using a questionnaire administered by volunteers. *British Medical Journal* 1990; **300**(6734):1253.

22 Chantrel J, Dugdill L,& Jeffrey V Exercise and leisure for older people. In Flanagan C & Barnes G (eds) *Health opportunities for older people in the North West*. A special report for the Regional Director of Public Health. University of Liverpool and North West Regional Task Force for Older People,1998.

23 Chaplin J Ageing Well Programme *Community Health Action* 1994; **34**:14–15.

24 *Parliament Hill surgery: a multidisciplinary clinic for the elderly*. Unpublished report, innovative primary care for older people in Camden and Islington project, 1999.

25 Poole J A health network to benefit over-65s. *Practice Nurse* 1998; **16**:487–91.

26 Rudd A, Martin SC, Hopper AH, *et al*. Community health care for South Asian Elders. *Health Visitor* 1997; **70**(5):182–4.

27 Morrell CJ, Walters SJ, Dixon S *et al*. Cost-effectiveness of community leg ulcer clinics: randomised control trial. *British Medical Journal* 1998; **316**:1487.

28 Gardner L Does nurse-led care mean second-class care? *Nursing Times* 1998; **94**(36):50–1.

29 Chambers N *Nurse practitioners in primary care*. Radcliffe Medical Press, Oxford 1998.

30 Full M, Walters S, Reid R, *et al.* An evaluation of a nurse-led ear care service in primary care: benefits and costs. *British Journal of General Practice* 1997; **47**:699–703.

31 See, for example, The appointment of health visitors as community health care co-ordinators in Birmingham City Social Services. Cited in Smith S *Health visitors working with older people*, p.29. CPHV, London 1997,or Rochdale district nurses providing a care management function for patients with complex nursing needs. Cited in *Memorandum by the Community and District Nursing Association to the Health Committee on the Relationship between Health and Social Services (HSS78) in the Health Committee First Report, Session 1998–99 Vol. II.* Minutes of Evidence and Appendices 74-II, The Stationery Office, London.

32 Harris W, Rivers P, & Goldstein R The potential role of community pharmacists in care management. *Health and Social Care in the Community* 1998; **6**(3):196–203.

33 Cumming M *Evaluation of the pilot district nurse care manager project.* Unpublished report, 1994.

34 Smith S Health visitors' working with older people, p.27. CPHVA 1997.

35 NHS Health Advisory Group *Services for people who are elderly: addressing the balance.* Section 443. The Stationery Office, London 1997.

36 Sumner P Primary concern: a specialist role with a fundholding practice. *Nursing Times* 1997; **93**(7):54–55.

37 Buxton V Freedom of choice: An integrated care scheme. *Nursing Times* 1996 ; **92**(43):57–59.

38 London Boroughs of Camden and Islington, The Camden and Islington Health Authority, and the Camden and Islington Community Trust *Joint operational policy for district nursing and home care services.* 1996.

39 Birmingham City Council Social Services Department and Birmingham Health Authorities and Trusts *The wavy line: homecare and community nursing working together.* 1994.

40 Audit Commission *First assessment review of district nursing services in England and Wales.* Audit Commission, London 1999.

41 Department of Health Note on charging arrangements for social care during the winter pressures initiative (HSS 25D): illustrative example in Middlesborough. Appendices to the First Report of the Health committee on the relationship between Health and Social Services: Session 1998–99. The Stationery Office, London.

42 Callahan S The RiTE stuff; homecare service for patients with chronic obstructive pulmonary disease. *Nursing Times* 1998; **94**(49):42–43.

43 Croxson B, Llewellyn L, Burdett K, *et al.* Home service. *Health Service Journal* 1998; 108:26–7.

44 Ministry of Health *A hospital plan for England and Wales.* HMSO, London 1962.

45 Armstrong A & Baker B. *An evaluation of the Lambeth Community Care Centre.* Lambeth, Southwark, & Lewisham Health Commission, London 1995.

46 North N & Hall D *First inner-city hospital: an appraisal of the first two years of operations*. Community Medicine and Nursing Research Unit, Paddington and North Kensington Health Authority, London 1984.

47 Eaton L. Arranged marriages: Grove Road GP practice case example. *Health Service Journal* 1998; **108**:24–6.

48 Williams J & Last A Intermediate care: smoothing the road to recovery. *Nursing Times* 1998; **94**(49):52–4.

49 Dawson S *Analysing organisations*. Macmillan Press, London 1992.

50 Petty Crewe M, Whatt I, & Sheldon T. Executive summary: A systematic review of the effectiveness of laxatives in the elderly. *Health Technology Assessment* 1997; **1**(13).

51 Kotter JP & Schlesinger LA Choosing strategies for Change. *Harvard Business Review.* 1979; **57**(2):106–14.

52 Lewin K *Field theory in social science*. Tavistock Publications, London 1952.

53 Moss Kanter R *The change masters*. Routledge, London 1985.

54 Alexander L D Successfully implementing strategic decisions. In Mayon-White B (ed) *Planning and managing change*. Open University, Buckingham 1986.

55 Cornwell J, *et al*. Leg ulcers: epidemiology and aetiology. *British Journal of Surgery* 1986; **73**(9):693–6.

56 Charles H The impact of leg ulcers on the patient's quality of life. *Professional nurse* 1995; **10**(9):571.

57 NHS Centre for Reviews and Dissemination , University of York Compression therapy for venous leg ulcers. *Effective Health Care Bulletin* 1997; **3**:4.

58 Harper D R, *et al*. Prevention of recurrence of venous ulceration: prospective randomised controlled trial over five years of class 2 and class 3 elastic compression. *Phlebology* 1995; **2**(1):872–3.

59 Bosanquet N Costs of venous ulcers: from maintenance therapy to investment programs. *Phlebology* 1992; **1**(1):44–6.

60 Audit Commission *First assessment: national report on district nursing services*. Audit Commission, London 1999.

61 Moffatt C & Stubbings N The Charing Cross approach to venous ulcers. *Nursing Standard.* 1990; **12**(10):6–9.

62 Moffatt CJ, Franks PJ, Oldroyd M, *et al*. Community clinics for leg ulcers and impact on healing. *British Medical Journal.* 1992; **305**(6866):1389–92.

63 See, for example, Training to improve nursing care of leg ulcers. *In NHS Executive Annual Report 1994/5*, p.36. Department of Health, London 1995; O'Hare L Implementing district-wide, nurse-led venous leg ulcers: a quality approach. *Journal of Wound Care* 1994; **3**(8):389–92; and Fogarty M Captain cuts ulcer teams leg work. *Medical Interface* 1996; **March**:58–9.

64 NHS Executive Letter *Improving clinical effectiveness*. Annexe B. EL(93) 115. Department of Health, London 1993.

65 Clinical Information Pack Number 1 *The management of leg ulcers in the community (with accompanying audit tool)*. Nursing Research and Development Unit, University of Liverpool.

66 Clinical Information Pack Number 1 The management of leg ulcers in the community (with accompanying audit tool). Nursing Research and Development Unit, University of Liverpool.

67 NHS Centre for Reviews and Dissemination, University of York Compression therapy for venous leg ulcers. *Effective Health Care Bulletin* 1997; **3**:4.

68 RCN Institute, Centre for Evidence-Based Nursing, University of York and the School of Nursing, Midwifery and Health Visiting, University of Manchester *Clinical practice guidelines: the management of patients with venous leg ulcers*. Royal College of Nursing, London 1998.

69 Morrell CJ, Walters SJ, Dixon S, *et al.* Cost-effectiveness of community leg ulcer clinics: randomised controlled trial. *British Medical Journal* 1998; **316**(7143):1487–91.

70 Audit Commission *First assessment: national report on district nursing services section 3*. Audit Commission, London 1999.

71 Harper D R, *et al.* (1995), op. cit.

72 Ruckley C Caring for patients with chronic leg ulcers: early specialist assessment offers the best hope of sustained healing [editorial]. *British Medical Journal* 1998; **316**: 7129.

73 Hamen C Patient perceptions of chronic leg ulcers. *Journal of Wound Care* 1994; **3**(2):99–101.

74 Department of Health *Modernising health and social services: national priorities guidance 1999/00–2001/02*. DOH, London 1998.

75 *Saving lives: our healthier nation*. Cm 4386. The Stationery Office, London 1999.

76 Department of Health *Health improvement programmes*. HSC/LAC 1998/167.

77 Department of Health *Modernising health and social services: national priorities guidance 1999/00–2001/02*, section 47. p. 14. DOH, London 1998.

78 Department of Health *Promoting independence: preventative strategies and support for adults*. Local authority circular (99)14. DOH, London 1999.

79 Department of Health *Caring about carers: a national strategy for carers*. LASSL (99)2. DOH, London 1999.

80 *Better services for vulnerable people – maintaining the momentum*. Annex B Action 1.

81 Audit Commission *The coming of age: improving care services for older people*. Audit Commission, London 1997.

82 Robinson J & Turnoch S Investing in rehabilitation. King's Fund, London 1998.

83 Dyke G The new NHS charter – a different approach. The Stationery Office, London 1998.

84 Department of Health *The long-term care charter*. The Stationery Office, London 1998.

85 Department of Health *Royal Commission on Long-term Care: with respect to old age.* Session 1998–99: Cm 4169. The Stationery Office, London 1999.

86 Department of Health *Modernising social services* The Stationery Office, London 1999.

87 Government response to the first report of the health committee on the relationship between health and social services. Session 1998–99: Cm 4320.

88 NHS Executive *A first-class service: quality in the NHS.* HSC 1998/113. The Stationery Office, London 1988.

89 NHS Executive *Quality and performance in the NHS: high-level performance indicators.* HSC 1999/999. The Stationery Office, London 1999.

INDEX